WOMEN'S GUIDE
TO FIGHTING
HEART DISEASE

"A very informative book, which I would recommend highly to all my women patients."

> —Maria A. deVilla, M.D., FACC, St. Joseph Health Center, Toronto

"If they use the advice of this book, women can really decrease their risk of having a heart attack. In the clearest, friendliest, most commonsensical manner, Dr. Helfant tells women what matters and why, and what to do about it."

> —Richard Berger, M.D., FACC, Past President, American Heart Association, Miami chapter

"Every woman can benefit from reading it."

> —Monte M. Bodenheimer, M.D., FACC, Director of Cardiology, Long Island Jewish Medical Center

"Deals with what every woman will most want and need to know: how really to take action for her health without being overwhelmed by all the unnecessary dos and don'ts."

> —Ronald S. Pennock, M.D., FACC, Clinical Professor of Medicine, Hahnemann University Hospital, Philadelphia

THE WOMEN'S GUIDE TO FIGHTING HEART DISEASE

Richard H. Helfant, M.D.

A Perigee Book

A Perigee Book
Published by The Berkley Publishing Group
200 Madison Avenue
New York, NY 10016

Grosset/Putnam edition: October 1993
First Perigee edition: November 1994

Library of Congress Cataloging-in-Publication Data
Helfant, Richard H.
[Women, take heart]
The women's guide to fighting heart disease / Richard H.
Helfant.
p. cm.
Originally published in 1993 under the title: Women, take
heart.
"A Perigee book."
Includes index.
ISBN 0-399-52141-0
1. Heart—Diseases.   2. Women—Diseases.
3. Heart—Diseases—Sex factors.   I. Title.
RC682.H394   1994
616.1′2′0082—dc20   94-11088   CIP

Book design: Rhea Braunstein

Printed in the United States of America
1 2 3 4 5 6 7 8 9 10

*To my mother, the first woman's heart I knew,
and to my miraculous children, Sharon and Steve,
who taught me what my own heart was all about*

Contents

Introduction

It is worse than folly not to recognize the truth. Everything has a moment when it can be remedied.
PEARL BUCK

Most women know that heart disease is the number-one killer in the United States—of men. Most women also realize the value of eating healthy food, exercising, and decreasing stress—for their families and other loved ones. Information is abundant, and readily available, in books, in newspapers and magazines, and on television and radio, about the risk of cardiovascular disease in men.

But the widespread belief that heart disease is exclusively a man's problem is a myth. Women—and most physicians—are not aware that cardiovascular disease is the number-one killer of women as well as men. The facts speak for themselves: Of the 520,000 people who die of heart attacks in the United States each year, almost half—about 250,000—are women. In addition, almost 100,000 women die of strokes. Substantially fewer women die annually from breast cancer (40,500) and lung cancer (41,500). Overall, heart and vascular diseases claim more American women's lives each year than do all forms of cancer combined.

Moreover, many of the factors that determine the risk of heart disease for women differ from those for men. Dr. William Castelli, a leading authority on heart disease and director of the Framingham Heart Study, which has done research on heart disease risk factors for forty years, has referred to these unique risks for women as a "whole new syndrome" associated with a "galloping progression of atherosclerosis." Women are largely unaware of the effects of estrogen, birth control pills, and cigarettes, and few know that if they smoke *and* take birth control pills they have about forty times more chance of heart disease than women who do not. Women above age thirty-five are particularly at risk. It is vital to understand the factors favoring heart disease, because they may be avoidable or modifiable. In fact, according to Dr. Dean Ornish, women may have to do less than men to affect their outlook positively. In a study he conducted evaluating the effect of life-style changes in reversing heart disease, women responded better than men, even when women did less to restrict their diets, exercise, or reduce stress. By understanding their risks and ways to minimize them, women can lessen the chances of being victims of what the American Heart Association has called "the silent epidemic."

My purpose in writing *The Women's Guide to Fighting*

Heart Disease is to help you change your perceptions about heart health. The book offers a simple, practical program to decrease heart disease risks in women without heart disease and to reduce the likelihood of recurrences in those of you who have an existing heart problem. The book also discusses heart disease itself: its causes and symptoms, tests and treatments for it, and their pros and cons. This information, which is based on my experience of what works for women, will give you insight into your circumstances and alternatives, so that you can communicate with your doctor in a more informed, satisfying way. The program in *The Women's Guide to Fighting Heart Disease* appreciates the fact that many of you have very busy schedules. It thus provides flexible methods to maximize heart health benefits in a minimum amount of time.

The purpose of developing and maintaining a healthy way of life for yourself as a woman is not only to decrease the risk of heart disease but also to feel well and feel good. Physical activity does not have to be strenuous to be beneficial. More women than ever are discovering that exercise in moderation is exhilarating. Healthy changes in eating do not have to be unduly restrictive. The food you eat *can* continue to be delicious and satisfying. By using simple new tools to maintain a healthy weight, you will decrease the chances of developing three big heart disease risks *and* discover a renewed sense of self at the same time.

Learning practical ways to identify and handle stress is vital to women's health today. Recent studies indicate a substantial increase in stress-related health problems among women. At work women have the same stress levels as men; but when they go home, men's levels fall, while women's remain high. There is also evidence that women handle stress in less healthy ways than men. This book suggests several techniques to decrease stress in your life, and thus improve your health and enhance your sense of vitality.

Women are often more concerned with caring for others than with caring for themselves. Since heart disease has been perceived as a male problem, some women may have difficulty motivating themselves to adopt a healthy life-style. When the facts about women and heart disease are made clear, and distinguished from the widespread myths, however, you will see that living a healthy life is as important for women as for men, and as easily attainable as it is rewarding.

This book provides a flexible approach that will enable you to discover that healthy living does not have to be yet another burden. It can be deeply satisfying. Adopting a healthy life-style means living well, being well, and once you make the adjustments part of your life, feeling well. This book encourages you to shape your own heart health program, in tune with your own preferences and circumstances. You will learn how to identify and understand your own strengths and weaknesses better, and how to build on the former and make allowances for the latter. The goal is not perfection but consistency, and realizing that your health benefits are achievable if you stay in alignment with your overall goals. The truth is that most of us, no matter how well motivated, slip at one time or another. This is part of being human, part of the learning process, and contrary to what you may have heard, it is no big deal. Eating an occasional gooey dessert, for instance, is not what causes health problems. The real danger involved in slipping is that you may be convinced you have failed and as a result may give up.

By taking control of your health practices, you will be

more able to take control of other aspects of your life. In so doing, you will achieve a greater sense of well-being, which is the true meaning of health. This is a marvelous opportunity for you personally. In addition, your new healthy living habits can be a model for family and friends. You thus may make a significant difference in their lives and health as well as your own.

To achieve the maximum benefit from reading *The Women's Guide to Fighting Heart Disease*, I suggest the following:

- Read through each chapter for an overview.
- Reread each chapter more closely, and this time imagine incorporating the material into your daily life. Picture specific situations in which you could apply the suggestions given and take action on your behalf.
- Think about the material actively, by assessing your circumstances and your strengths and weaknesses. Set your priorities, and pick and choose among your alternatives.
- Earmark the pages and special sections or lists that are most important to you. Make notes in the margins or on a pad. Underline or highlight. Make the book a companion and a resource to consult for valuable reminders. If you've borrowed the book from a friend or a library, take notes on what's relevant for you.
- Do the exercises and write your action plan as instructed in the "Taking Action" and "Getting Started" sections. These are logical ways to cross the threshold from reading to doing, and are vital to your success.
- Take a few minutes each day to reflect on where you are, as outlined in the "Recording Your Progress" sections. Doing so will help you evaluate your plan, spot any pitfalls,

and learn from your experiences. Do this every day for four to six weeks.

  • Refer now and then to the "To Sum Up" sections at the end of chapters, for a refresher course.

  • As you read the book and, moreover, when you apply its principles, keep in mind the wise words of Hillel: "If I am not for myself, then who will be for me? If not now, when?"

THE
WOMEN'S GUIDE
TO FIGHTING
HEART DISEASE

CHAPTER 1

Women and Heart Disease: The Silent Epidemic

The coronary heart disease epidemic among women is real. . . . Changing life-style to prevent heart disease is as relevant for women as for men.
ROSE STAMLER, NORTHWESTERN UNIVERSITY

The American woman is at risk of developing coronary disease and requires evaluation. And women must know this.
NANETTE KASS WENGER, M.D.

Why has the American Heart Association called the truth about heart disease among women "the silent epidemic"? Some of the chief reasons:

First, more American women die each year of cardiovascular disease than of breast cancer, uterine cancer, and lung cancer combined. To put it into perspective: Women have a 1 in 9 risk of developing breast cancer—the same risk a woman between the ages of forty-five and sixty-four has of suffering cardiovascular disease. But when a woman reaches sixty-five, her risk of heart disease climbs to 1 in 3.

Dr. Elizabeth Barrett-Connor has summarized the matter: "The magnitude of the problem of heart disease in women is so much greater than [that of other diseases] women and science have been worried about. This is not appreciated by the female public."

Second, women are less likely than men to survive a heart attack. Statistics indicate that women who have heart attacks are twice as likely as men to die from them. The reasons for this are not clear, but according to *The New England Journal of Medicine*, "Women who are hospitalized for coronary heart disease undergo fewer major diagnostic and therapeutic procedures than men." A recent study of 1,659 women and 3,232 men who had had heart attacks showed that fewer women than men had thrombolytic, or "clot buster," therapy (14 versus 26 percent); catheterization (40 versus 58 percent); or balloon angioplasty (14 versus 22 percent).

Third, the diagnostic and therapeutic procedures for coronary heart disease are less accurate and less reliable for women than for men. The standard treadmill stress test, for example, is less accurate for women; although this has been known for years, the reason remains a mystery. The risks associated with coronary bypass surgery are significantly higher for women than for men, and balloon angioplasty, by which blocked coronary arteries are opened with a balloon, is less effective for women. In addition, complications from taking thrombolytic medications are more frequent in women than in men.

The risk factors that determine heart disease differ in many respects between women and men. For the most part, women were omitted from the large trials in the 1980s that evaluated the effects of reducing certain risk factors on the development of heart disease. Many physicians have assumed that the results of those studies apply equally to men and women.

More recent research, however, indicates a heart disease risk factor profile "for women only." Smoking is more of a risk factor for women than for men. The Framingham Heart Study has shown that a fifty-five-year-old woman smoker is in more danger of having a heart attack than a fifty-five-year-old man who smokes. Despite this, fewer women are kicking the habit than men. Obesity and diabetes too appear to play a more important role in determining women's risk of heart disease than men's. Evidence from the Arizona Heart Institute shows that a diabetic woman with heart disease is more likely to die of a heart attack than a diabetic man with heart disease. The role of birth control pills and estrogen, and of menopause, as risk factors have not been emphasized sufficiently to women, and the advantages and disadvantages of estrogen replacement therapy to reduce the risk of heart disease in postmenopausal women have not been studied adequately.

Is there any good news amid this startling array of facts about women and heart disease? Fortunately, as mentioned in the introduction, the answer is a resounding yes. Many if not most of women's risk factors for heart disease can be modified. And according to Dr. Dean Ornish's research on reversing heart disease, women actually may have to do less than men to affect their outlook favorably.

SYMPTOMS: CHEST DISCOMFORT AND SHORTNESS OF BREATH

A major concern related to women and heart disease is in the interpretation of symptoms such as chest discomfort and shortness of breath. It is vital that women—and their physicians—take these symptoms seriously. Phyllis, a woman referred to me by her internist, is a case in point:

Like most women, Phyllis had no idea that she was at risk for heart disease. She suddenly began to experience severe shortness of breath walking from her car in the parking lot to her office building, and as she later told me, "I just assumed that it was because I was sixty-two years old, overweight, out of shape, and a two-pack-a-day smoker." After several days, her problem worsened. Frightening chest pains began to accompany these episodes, causing Phyllis to stop in the middle of the parking lot before continuing to the office.

Phyllis's internist examined her and reassured her that the symptoms were probably due to emotional stress, and he gave her a prescription for a tranquilizer. The pills did nothing to relieve her symptoms. One night she woke up gasping for breath, and with severe pains in her chest. Her husband took her to the hospital, where she was told she was having a heart attack.

After four days Phyllis seemed to be doing well, and she was moved out of the coronary care unit. On day six, however, while strolling in a hospital corridor, she became short of breath and felt pressure in her chest. Her internist was not sure whether this was the result of emotional stress or a heart problem. This time Phyllis insisted on getting another opinion, and I was asked to see her. It was clear to me that Phyllis needed further study immediately, and so an angiogram was performed. The test revealed that Phyllis had a 90-percent blockage in the coronary artery responsible for her heart attack and now the artery was threatening to close completely. We were able to dilate the artery with balloon angioplasty, and consequently Phyllis's symptoms disappeared. After being discharged from the hospital, she quit smoking and lost twenty pounds, and she is still doing very well. Phyllis is living proof of how women must heed their symptoms, as must their physicians. Clearly, Phyllis was right to ask for a second opinion. She was aware of her symptoms, and relied on informed communication with her doctors.

The most common initial symptom of heart disease in women is the chest discomfort of angina pectoris. This is not, as many think, experienced as a true pain, but usually is described as tightness, pressure, heaviness, squeezing, or constriction in the center of the chest. One sufferer described it by saying: "It feels like an elephant sitting on my chest." This discomfort is caused by a decrease in the amount of oxygen going to the heart muscle through one or more blocked coronary arteries, which supply oxygen to the heart. Chest discomfort is diagnosed as angina pectoris when the characteristic symptoms are provoked by physical activity (as it was in Phyllis's case). The symptoms last from two to thirty minutes, typically ten to fifteen. When the physical activity is stopped, the chest discomfort disappears within minutes.

The first sign of coronary heart disease varies among individual women. This discomfort may start in the shoulders (more frequently the left), or spread there from the center of the chest, and then move down the arms or into the neck or jaw. Sudden, unusual shortness of breath, either alone or accompanying chest tightness, may arise during ordinary physical activity that did not cause difficulty in the past. Less commonly, symptoms of angina pectoris can be brought on by emotional upset and exposure to cold, especially after a heavy meal.

Whatever the onset of symptoms, it is vital to heed

these warning signs of potential heart disease and to consult your physician without delay. Early diagnosis and appropriate treatment may reduce the risks and eventually prevent a heart attack. If you have symptoms that sound like these, discuss them in detail with your physician. Do not be too intimidated or frightened to ask specific and appropriate questions: Do my symptoms suggest the possibility of heart disease? If so, why—what characteristics suggest that they do? If not, why not? The answers should be based on the nature of the symptoms themselves, not on secondary factors such as your risk, emotional state, life circumstances, and so on.

STRESS TESTS AND CORONARY ARTERIOGRAPHY

After evaluating your symptoms, most physicians will take an electrocardiogram (ECG or EKG). A normal ECG is a pretty good indication that there is no significant heart damage, but does not necessarily mean there is no problem. It is important to assess how your heart performs during the stress of physical activity. This can be done with a stress ECG test or a stress thallium test. Both are performed by having you walk on a treadmill while hooked up to an ECG monitor. The speed and slope of the treadmill are increased gradually, until a targeted heart rate is reached—unless significant chest discomfort or shortness of breath occurs, in which case the test is stopped. The ECG is then evaluated for characteristic changes that might point to a possible heart problem. Overall, the stress ECG test is about 65 percent accurate. Among women there are more false positive results, however, meaning that the results suggest heart disease, when in fact there is no problem.

For this reason, a thallium stress test is done often on women instead of the stress ECG or after a positive stress ECG. The thallium test proceeds like the ECG, with a monitor and treadmill. At the end of the treadmill exercise, a small amount of thallium, a radioactive compound, is injected into a vein. A special camera takes pictures that reveal any areas of the heart that have not taken up the thallium. These "cold spots" indicate a high likelihood of blockage of the coronary arteries supplying the area with oxygen. The thallium stress test is about 85 percent accurate in diagnosing coronary artery disease—20 percent more accurate than the stress ECG; it is also considerably more expensive than the stress ECG. Normal (i.e., negative) results on a stress ECG test usually mean you have been screened adequately for serious coronary artery disease. But if the stress ECG is positive, the thallium stress test will determine more precisely whether or not a significant problem exists.

If your symptoms or the results from one of the stress tests suggest strongly that you have coronary artery disease *and* that the problem may be severe, you are probably a candidate for coronary arteriography, also referred to as heart catheterization. In this procedure, a long, thin tube is threaded through an artery in the arm or groin and into the coronary arteries. A dye is injected into them and X-ray pictures are taken. This is ordinarily not a painful procedure, but it does require going to a hospital. Coronary arteriography is usually safe; while complications can occur, they are rare. The main reason for having coronary arteriography is that it is the most accurate way to determine whether or not you have coronary artery disease (blocked coronary arteries), how many of the three major coronary arteries have significant blockages, and what needs to be done. On the basis of this invaluable X-ray "road map" of the coronary arteries, a judgment can be made as to whether treatment with medication, balloon angioplasty, or bypass surgery is warranted.

If your physician suggests any tests, ask the specific purpose of each test. Is it to clarify the diagnosis, to assess the severity of the problem, or what? How accurate is each test, and what are its advantages and disadvantages? What is the particular relevance or value of each test for women?

If your physician does not think tests are needed, ask why. Is the diagnosis totally clear? If so, on what objective basis? An appropriate answer might be: "Your chest discomfort has none of the characteristics of angina pectoris. It lasts only seconds [or hours, rather than minutes] and is not in the typical locations. And your symptoms of discomfort are not typical of angina pectoris; they are not brought on by physical activity." It makes sense to ascertain that there is absolutely no doubt that you do not have a coronary artery problem.

Your questions merit concrete, specific answers, and—it bears repeating—it is essential that you establish open communication with your physician. Remember that you are talking about your heart and your health and what you are *entitled* to know. Some of my patients find it helpful to write out questions in advance, so they don't freeze once they're in my office. Whatever means you use, this type of communication is the best way to establish a relationship with your physician based on mutual trust and respect.

HEART ATTACK

The discomfort of a heart attack is more intense than angina. Typically, it is experienced as a crushing sensation in the center of the chest. The discomfort lasts longer than angina—usually more than an hour. If untreated, it may go on for several hours, usually varying in intensity during that time. Sweating, shortness of breath, nausea and vomiting, and dizziness or faintness frequently accompany a heart attack.

The symptoms of a heart attack always constitute a medical emergency. If you suspect you are having an attack, you must go to the nearest hospital emergency room, as soon as possible. Do not delay, in hope that the discomfort will pass. Call a rescue squad if one is available in your community, and if not, have someone drive you to the hospital; do not attempt to drive yourself. The staff at the hospital emergency room will alert your doctor to meet you there if necessary. It is critical to get to the hospital immediately, because the risk of dying from a heart attack is highest in the very first hours after an attack. In addition, thrombolytic ("clot buster") therapy, which can open up blocked coronary arteries rapidly and reduce the amount of heart damage, is effective only in those first few hours after an attack.

Of course, not all chest discomfort originates from the heart, and false alarms do occur. Yet it is always better to err on the side of caution and seek medical attention for an unusual episode of particularly oppressive, crushing chest discomfort. Tell the emergency room personnel that you are experiencing severe chest pains. They should give you prompt attention; if they do not, be persistent with physicians or nurses. They can quickly do an ECG and blood tests to differentiate accurately between a heart attack and a false alarm.

REDUCING THE RISKS OF HEART DISEASE

In addition to taking such symptoms as chest discomfort and shortness of breath seriously, it is important for women actively to reduce their risks of developing heart disease. As research has begun, albeit belatedly, to focus on these risks, significant information has emerged. Low levels of "good," or HDL, cholesterol (less than 40 milligrams/deciliter), together with high levels of lipids called triglycerides (more than 150–250 mg/dl), are a red flag for heart disease risk in women. (For a more complete understanding of "good" and "bad" cholesterol and triglycerides, see chapter 5.) Women with low HDL and high triglyceride levels tend to have elevated blood sugar and high blood pressure. According to Dr. William Castelli of the Framingham Heart Study, they will end up with a "galloping progression of atherosclerosis, even though their total cholesterol is 190 or 210." Most authorities feel that, in contrast (on the basis of studies mainly on men), maintaining a total cholesterol level below 200 is sufficient to lower the risk of heart disease.

Obviously, total cholesterol levels alone are not adequate for assessing a woman's heart disease risk. Women with high HDL levels, for example, have a *lower* risk of heart disease even when their total cholesterol is somewhat elevated. It is important for women to have their HDL and triglyceride levels checked in addition to their total cholesterol, especially since the methods for correcting low HDL cholesterol and elevated triglycerides are very different from those for lowering total cholesterol.

Before menopause, women have a significantly lower risk of coronary artery disease than men. Physicians have long believed that estrogen is responsible for this premenopausal protection. However, the potential role of estrogen replacement to prevent heart disease in postmenopausal women is not clear-cut. Studies have shown that women who undergo estrogen replacement therapy after menopause do decrease their risk of heart disease by as much as one-third to one-half, and estrogen replacement has reduced the risk of osteoporosis (the bone loss that may also afflict postmenopausal women) and postmenopausal symptoms for many women. But there is potential risk associated with estrogen replacement: taking estrogen may *increase* the risk of uterine and breast cancer.

The relevance of estrogen was made clear to Doris, a forty-six-year-old woman who was sent to me for an evaluation of her chest pains. The nature of her symptoms strongly suggested coronary artery disease, but even though she was a two-pack-a-day smoker, she seemed rather young to have a heart problem. As we started the physical examination, Doris told me, "I don't know if this means anything, but I had a hysterectomy when I was twenty-five because of fibroids." This *was* an important part of the story, because the hormone changes resulting from a hysterectomy are similar to menopausal changes and cause women to rapidly lose their protection against heart disease. Fortunately for Doris, the tests showed only one blockage in a minor artery. She stopped smoking and her chest pains soon subsided.

Studies on estrogen and its reduction of heart disease risk have shown that about half of its protective effect comes from its ability to increase HDL cholesterol levels. It is known that women under age fifty have higher levels of this good cholesterol and lower levels of bad (LDL) cholesterol than men. These levels change dramatically after menopause, and that change coincides with a striking increase in coronary artery disease. "After menopause, it takes women only six to ten years to catch up to men," says Dr. Castelli. In Doris's case, simply giving up cigarettes was enough to boost her good cholesterol to a normal level.

The benefits of estrogen replacement in lowering the risk of coronary artery disease must be weighed carefully against the increased risk of uterine and breast cancer, a risk that varies among women. If you have a personal or family history of such cancer, it is prudent to avoid estrogen replacement. On the other hand, if you have had a hysterectomy, uterine cancer is no longer a concern. If you have a significant risk of coronary artery disease, you might consider low-dose estrogen replacement. If you already have coronary heart disease, you may be interested in two recent studies which reported that women with heart disease live longer after receiving estrogen replacement therapy. The large-scale Woman's Health Initiative, recently begun under the sponsorship of the National Institutes of Health and its former director, Dr. Bernadine Healy, is conducting a study on estrogen. The Postmenopausal Estrogen/Progestin Intervention project should provide more precise information in this area. I suggest you consult with your doctor about the pluses and minuses of estrogen therapy as they apply to you.

Women who take oral contraceptives have a higher risk of heart attack than those who do not. But since the overall likelihood for most healthy young women to have a heart attack is small, the risk from oral contraceptives is minor. That is, unless a woman smokes. If you smoke *and* use oral contraceptives, you are about forty times more likely to have a heart attack and up to twenty-two times more likely to have a stroke than women who do not. This is particularly true for women thirty-five years old and older. In view of the dramatic increase in the risk of heart disease caused by the combination of taking oral contraceptives and smoking, the message is very clear: *If you use oral contraceptives, quit smoking.* If you just can't quit, change to another form of contraception.

There are other risks associated with smoking and using oral contraceptives, as the following example illustrates. Debbie, thirty-four years old, came to the hospital emergency room complaining of episodes of severe shortness of breath over several days. Despite her considerable difficulty breathing, a physical exam, an ECG, and blood tests showed no evidence of a heart attack. It was obvious that Debbie was very ill, though, and I was asked to see her. In talking to her, I learned that she had been a heavy smoker since her teens and had always used birth control pills for contraception. She also told me that she had had some recent discomfort in her left leg. The information she gave me led to the diagnosis.

Debbie had developed a blood clot (phlebitis) in her left leg. Pieces of the clot periodically were breaking off and traveling up to her lungs, where they lodged (what is known in medical terminology as a pulmonary embolism) and caused the severe shortness of breath. Like heart attacks, blood clots are common in women who smoke and take oral contraceptives. Debbie was treated with anticoagulants, or "blood thinners," and she made a rapid recovery—and vowed to quit smoking when she was discharged from the hospital.

AGE, RISK, AND PREVENTION

Your need to determine the presence of risk factors for heart disease and to take preventive measures is related to how old you are. The onset of menopause (usually around age fifty) is a most important time for evaluation. Hysterectomy is a cardiovascular equivalent of menopause, since both result in decreased estrogen levels.

Before age 35

1. Have your weight, blood pressure, and cholesterol/triglyceride levels measured.

2. Do not smoke and use oral contraceptives. If you use oral contraceptives, quit smoking. If you can't quit, choose another form of contraceptive.

Ages 35–50

1. In addition to the weight, blood pressure, and cholesterol/triglyceride profiles, have a blood sugar test and a routine electrocardiogram.

2. Do not smoke and use oral contraceptives. Your risk of cardiovascular disease is forty times higher than in women who do not smoke and use oral contraceptives.

3. If you smoke and/or are overweight, quit smoking and develop healthy eating habits. These life-style changes are especially urgent if your blood pressure and/or blood sugar are at all high, or if there is a strong history of high blood pressure, diabetes, or heart disease in your family.

4. Begin a physical activity and stress reduction program.

02/07/98   21:15   H   A7   6867
REFUNDS WITHIN 30 DAYS WITH RECEIPT ONLY
NON-RETAIL SALES ARE FINAL

PUBLISHER	CROWN	CROWN
PRICE	SAVINGS	PRICE

ACROSS THE RIVER & INTO
ST 7700 060515008   10%   6.30
WORDS OF FIGHTING MEN
18 41700 039962410   10%   9.90
HOW WILLIAMS
NA 21.95 041624968   (80%)   18.35
SUBTOTAL   34.55
SALES TAX @ 6.00%   2.49
TOTAL   36.29
TENDERED CHARGE   36.29
5463032522601833 MAYBE APPROVAL 093402

YOUR SAVINGS AT CROWN... $ 6.29

SUPER CROWN #152

12/09/94   21:15   H   47   6933
REFUNDS WITHIN 30 DAYS WITH RECEIPT ONLY
MAGAZINE SALES ARE FINAL!

PUBLISHER PRICE	CROWN SAVINGS	CROWN PRICE
ACROSS THE RIVER & INTO		
1@ 7.00 0020519206	10%	6.30
WOMENS GT FIGHTING HEAR		
1@ 11.00 0399521410	10%	9.90
HANK WILLIAMS		
1@ 22.95 0316249866	20%	18.36
SUBTOTAL	$	34.56
SALES TAX @ 5.00%	$	1.73
TOTAL	$	36.29
TENDERED CHARGE	$	36.29

5420392228019339 04/96 APPROVAL 009482

YOUR SAVINGS AT CROWN... $ 6.39

After age 50 (postmenopausal)

1. Have your weight, blood pressure, cholesterol/triglyceride levels, and blood sugar measured, and have an electrocardiogram.

2. Quit smoking and develop healthy eating habits, if you have not done so already.

3. Gradually initiate a program of physical activity.

4. Incorporate the tools to defuse stresses in your life.

TO SUM UP

1. Cardiovascular disease is the number-one killer of women as well as men in the United States. It claims more women's lives each year than all forms of cancer combined. The diagnostic and therapeutic procedures for coronary artery disease are not as accurate or reliable for women as for men.

2. The factors that determine the risk of heart disease differ in many respects between women and men. A unique profile has been identified as a signal for elevated risk in women: a combination of low good (HDL) cholesterol and high triglycerides constitutes this profile. Total cholesterol levels alone are not enough for assessing a woman's risk of heart disease. In addition, smoking and being overweight pose more of a risk in women than in men.

3. Before menopause, women have a substantially lower risk of coronary artery disease than men. Estrogen may be responsible for this protection. However, premenopausal women who smoke and use oral contraceptives are about forty times more likely to have a heart attack than those who do not.

4. The most common initial symptom of coronary artery disease in women is the chest discomfort of angina pectoris. Early diagnosis can be made with a stress electrocardiogram or a stress thallium test. If there is a suspicion of severe disease, coronary arteriography, or heart catheterization, may be required.

5. If you experience the crushing chest pain that suggests a heart attack, it is essential that you go immediately to the nearest hospital. While it may be a false alarm, it is always better to err on the side of caution and seek medical attention.

CHAPTER 2

Mind-Body Communication: The Hidden Force for Health

I think, therefore I am.
RENÉ DESCARTES

*Thoughts in your mind have made you what
you are, and thoughts in your mind will make
you what you become.*
GERALDINE PONDER

The power of the mind to affect the body is undeniable. One of the first experiences to teach me the importance of a positive approach to health and longevity involved a wonderful patient named Brenda. She had been having severe, progressive, prolonged anginal chest pains, which rapidly became unstable and unresponsive to medication. By the time she came to the hospital, she was at very high risk for heart bypass surgery because of extensive heart damage and widespread coronary artery blockage. Yet despite the risk, surgery seemed the only possibility. I had become attached to her and was worried that she would not make it. On the night before her surgery, I went to the coronary care unit to visit her. I was making idle conversation, when after several minutes, Brenda looked straight into my eyes and said, "Don't worry, Doc. I'm going to sail through this operation. A lot of people depend on me, and I've got a lot to do before I'm finished with this life!" She did "sail through" the surgery, and ten years later she still was kidding me about how nervous I had been that night.

The power of the mind to affect the body holds true for men as well as women. Mark, my best friend in medical school, "knew" he was going to die of a heart attack before age forty. The idea obsessed him. When I would say, "Look, you can't possibly 'know,'" Mark would answer quietly, "I do know." During our second year in medical school, his father told him he had had pain in his left shoulder while playing handball. Mark, who had yet to see a patient in his medical training, tried to reassure his father that it was nothing. Two weeks later, his father suddenly fell over while playing handball and died, at age sixty. I was with Mark on the night when he received the news; it devastated him. From that night on he "knew." One night, while jogging with a medical colleague, *he* suddenly fell over and died, at age thirty-nine. I have known many patients like Mark, both men and women, whose intense guilt, while often repressed, leads to an absolute belief about their future health and longevity. This belief is so powerful that it becomes a self-fulfilling prophecy.

Many years ago, I began to sense a change in attitude in some of my patients on the day before their heart surgery. Most of my patients, freely admitting their anxieties about the surgery, regarded it as an unpleasant but necessary hurdle to get over in order to get on with their lives.

But in others, there seemed to be an air of resignation. Even when they did not have a bad surgical risk, these patients frequently did not do well; sometimes they did not survive the operation. I decided to talk to these seemingly resigned patients before their surgery. "You don't think you're going to make it, do you?" I would say. After a startled look they would usually acknowledge it, and then all sorts of things would come rushing out. Women would often express profound feelings of guilt ("My mother died at sixty-two. I'm sixty-eight and I've outlived her") and of not deserving to live ("I've provided for my family and my children are grown. I've done what I needed to do"); they would reveal unresolved personal conflicts ("My daughter is hooked on drugs, and I don't know what to do. If only I had been a better mother") and job-related tension ("I hate my job, but with my husband's income, I can't quit"). I canceled surgery for these patients until we were able to work on their problems.

Sometimes an unexpected turn of events would change a patient's outcome dramatically, as in the case of Cheryl, an obese, chain-smoking lawyer who did what she wanted, whenever and wherever she wanted. Two days after a massive heart attack, while in the coronary care unit, she blithely resumed her three-pack-a-day smoking habit, despite the CCU rules *and* the risk to her life. After several attempts at politely telling her, through the fog of her smoke-filled room, that she was still very unstable and was in danger of not making it, I lost my temper at her continuing to ignore me. In desperation I blurted out, "We care about you, we're trying to save your life, but you don't seem to care. This is a team effort, and that includes you. If you aren't willing to cooperate and just want to kill yourself by smoking, you don't need us or anyone else!"

Cheryl looked coldly right through me and said, "Nobody talks to me like that. I want you to leave my room!" Later that afternoon, as I pondered Cheryl's situation, one of the CCU nurses came into my office and exclaimed, "She's stopped smoking!"

A year later, Cheryl had kicked the habit and had lost sixty pounds. I finally felt comfortable enough to ask her what remarkable revelation she had had in the CCU that day that had almost certainly saved her life. Her answer: "No thanks to you and your lousy bedside manner, Doc. I simply decided I liked being around." Cheryl continued to take good care of herself and do remarkably well. When thoughts or feelings change in this manner, they can have a significant impact on the course of a patient's illness—no matter what the doctor's bedside manner!

Physicians throughout history have known the importance of the mind in both harming, causing illness, and in healing. Modern-day knowledge of disease physiology and advances in medical technology have led many doctors to disregard the role of the mind. But recent studies relying on more objective methods have demonstrated the significance of the mind-body relationship. If they were not already aware, doctors are waking up to the fact that the mind has substantial influence on health and disease.

My experience has convinced me that all of us, men and women alike, have a deep-seated sense of our own well-being; this in turn creates an underlying expectation about our present and future health which profoundly affects how healthy we are and even how long we will live. Our state of mind can be mobilized as an invaluable complement to modern medical treatment. Good medical care and the mind form a powerful team, one reinforcing the other. This does not mean that the mind alone can cure illness. Using only part of our health arsenal, as some proponents of "alternative medicine" advocate, makes no sense. Likewise, the power of the mind is not to be readily dismissed, as some high tech–oriented physicians would have it. Consider some recent evidence that state of mind has a direct bearing on cardiovascular illness:

A study conducted at Stanford showed that behavioral change can prevent repeated heart attacks. More than a thousand heart attack survivors were taught specifically to modify their hostile behavior. After four years of behavior modification classes, they were compared with survivors who took classes on medical risks alone. Even when their heart conditions were similar, those who were taught to modify their behavior and relax more proved fifty percent more likely to survive.

The men in the study who did not exhibit hostile behavior had fewer repeated heart attacks. On the other hand, the women scoring low in exhibiting hostility were more apt to die from a repeated heart attack, even though their physical condition was similar to the men's. According to Stanford psychologist Carl Thoreson, "Depression may be what's going on here. The women may be turning anger inward—onto themselves." This study points out that women who are programmed to be "nice" can be under greater stress when being "good." They need to release some of their anger to be relieved of stress (see chapter 4). Two other significant risk factors were found for these women: having more than two children and working in clerical jobs. These seemingly unrelated aspects may have as their common ingredient the loss of power and control.

In another study, this one at Harvard, yearly health surveys were correlated with psychological tests. Subjects who rated highest on a "life satisfaction" scale had one-tenth the rate of serious illness of those who were most dissatisfied. These findings were statistically independent of the effects of smoking, obesity, and genetics.

A woman's style of coping may have an important influence on her health. There are, of course, various ways of dealing with life circumstances and stress, and among those that have been studied are: intrusive positive thought, namely, positive admonitions and self-talk; intrusive negative thought (as in self-blame, criticism, perfectionistic tendencies, catastrophic or irrational thinking); avoidance, as in minimizing the significance of a problem or not dwelling on a stressful situation; and problem-focused coping, behavioral attempts to change environmental stresses or one's own behavior. Women with a minimum of positive thoughts and problem-focused behavior usually have an excess of negative thoughts and avoid dealing with stressful situations. This unhealthy behavior often leads to stress-related illnesses.

Another coping behavior that researchers have identified is something they call "hardiness." This consists of a sense of commitment rather than alienation toward work and life; a sense of personal internal control over life circumstances; and a sense that changes in life are challenges rather than threats. In a number of studies, individuals with hardy appraisals of work and life remain physically healthier, particularly when they are experiencing a great deal of stress.

TAKING ACTION

The purpose of this exercise is to provide you with an awareness of the thoughts and feelings you have about your health and health habits. Simply by answering the questions below, you may feel your negative, self-defeating thoughts and feelings about your health begin to loosen their hold, as your positive thoughts and feelings begin to be reinforced. Those negative ideas are not necessarily facts about the way you are or the way it has to be; they are just thoughts and feelings and do not have to control you. You can simply become aware of them if you have them, but equally aware that you can make a conscious choice to change them at any time.

This exercise should take about ten minutes. Write your answers to the following:

1. How much impact do you think *changing* your health habits would have on your health outlook? (a) a lot (b) very little (c) don't know
   Why?
2. Do you see any point in evaluating your thoughts and feelings about your health? (a) yes (b) no (c) don't know
3. Would any changes or events in your life cause you to evaluate your thoughts and feelings about your health and your health habits? (a) yes (b) no (c) don't know
4. Where do you think your beliefs about your health and your health habits came from? (a) parents (b) just "a sense" (c) other (specify) (d) don't know
5. Is there any factual basis for these beliefs? (a) yes (b) not really (c) don't know
6. Do you believe that studies showing that more posi-

tive attitudes promote health apply to you? (a) yes (b) no (c) don't know

If not, why not?

7. Do you believe that studies showing the benefits of good health habits apply to you? (a) yes (b) no (c) don't know

If not, why not?

8. Do you think your beliefs about your health and health habits could be faulty? (a) yes (b) no (c) don't know

If not, why not?

9. Do you feel you are entitled to take good care of yourself so that you can enhance your own health and well-being? (a) yes (b) no (c) don't know

If not, why not?

10. Make three columns on a piece of paper. In the left column write five thoughts or feelings that do *not* serve your health. In the center column list corresponding alternatives that would serve your health. In the right column indicate ("yes" or "no") whether or not you are willing to make a commitment to the alternative that would serve your health.

HOW TO INTERPRET YOUR ANSWERS

1. The answer (b) to questions 1, 2, 3, 6, 7, and 9 indicates a sense of resignation. I suggest you read further, to appreciate better that you need not view your current and future health as inevitable. You are entitled to take good care of yourself, and if you do, you can make a big difference in your life.

2. If you answered (a) to questions 1, 2, 3, 6, 7, and 9, you demonstrate a positive attitude about taking control of your health. This will serve you well, and the rest of this book will help you build on your positive attitude with a sound health program.

3. If the majority of your answers were "don't know," you apparently have not given much thought to this subject previously. As you read on, perhaps you will see that there is a great deal you can do to live a long, healthy, fulfilling life.

A POTENTIAL PITFALL

There is only one pitfall in this chapter—*not* doing the written exercise! I encourage you to do it and to review your answers. If you think about the questions and read your answers with an open mind, you may gain valuable insights into yourself and your beliefs that will improve your views about living a healthy and rewarding life. Since your thoughts and feelings about being fulfilled and healthy determine your health habits, it is vital that you understand your own view of your health. The worst thing that can happen is nothing: you will have "wasted" several minutes of your time. On the other hand, this exercise can provide you with an awareness that could change your entire view of your health and your life. The discovery that you really are worth it and that taking good care of yourself is important is the first step to a more satisfying, healthy life and a healthy heart.

TO SUM UP

1. Recent studies have confirmed what physicians always have known: that the mind has a substantial influence on health and disease.

2. These studies indicate that certain behaviors and states of mind profoundly affect the risk of serious illness and the chances for long-term survival among heart attack victims.

3. Developing an awareness of your thoughts and feelings about your health may enhance your power to develop good health habits. Further, becoming aware of any negative, self-defeating thoughts and feelings you may have about your health may be a step toward resisting them and reinforcing positive thoughts and feelings.

4. Studies evaluating styles of coping with stress—positive or negative thought processes, avoidance, focusing on problems—have identified a relationship between individuals' coping styles and their health.

5. It is vital for you to be aware of your health, and your attitude toward your health. Recognizing that you are worth taking care of is the first move to a more fulfilling, healthy life and a healthy heart.

CHAPTER 3

Physical Activity: The Great Health Facilitator

Opportunities are usually disguised . . . so most people don't recognize them.
ANN LANDERS

The journey of a thousand miles begins with a single step.
LAO-TZU

Physical activity is the best first step to health. It is the most direct way for you to discover, or rediscover, the wonder of your body. It allows you to experience vitality and provides an immediate sense of control of your body's health and well-being. In addition to having its own inherent benefits, physical activity is a great physical and mental health facilitator, and wonderfully regenerative. Your senses come alive and are attuned more delicately when you engage in regular physical activity.

There is good news about actually doing physical activity. Research has shown that women can obtain its major health benefits with a minimum of effort and in a minimum of time. The old myths of "no pain, no gain" and of long-distance jogging as the way to become invulnerable to cardiovascular disease finally have been put into proper perspective. Evidence shows that women can enjoy the benefits of physical activity with the equivalent of walking half an hour a day, four days a week.

The Institute for Aerobics Research in Texas evaluated the fitness levels of more than 3,000 women and followed their progress for eight years. While the sedentary women did have a mortality rate substantially higher than that of the more fit women, the principal benefits of physical activity came even after very little physical activity. Women who simply walked an average of thirty minutes a day decreased their risk of heart disease almost by half.

The American Heart Association recently stated that a sedentary life-style is a risk factor for heart disease comparable to smoking, cholesterol abnormalities, and high blood pressure. It pointed out also that low-intensity physical activity, performed regularly, can lower the risk of heart disease.

As Dr. Edward Cooper, president of the organization, noted: "For years, the American Heart Association has emphasized aerobic exercise . . . three to four times a week for thirty minutes to an hour. . . . Any physical exercise is better than none. Housework, gardening, shuffleboard—anything that causes us to move—is beneficial."

Besides mind-body communication (discussed in chapter 2), it is important to recognize the reverse, body-mind communication. In mind-body communication, the mind sends ongoing messages to the body and thus affects its health and well-being. In body-mind communication, the body sends *its* ongoing messages to the mind. Each influences the other continuously, in positive or negative ways. Physical activity, then, provides a powerful entry into this cycle through the body.

When women have a vague sense of discomfort in the body, there is a certain level of physical tension. The blood vessels tend to be constricted and the flow of blood becomes sluggish. Consequently, there is an underlying feeling of tension, constriction, and sluggishness. Physical activity is a unique—and simple—way to release muscle and body tension, and open up arteries to increase the flow of blood through the body. When, through exercise, you rediscover your body and become comfortable with it, you have a physical sense of health and of your self. This heightened physical sensation translates to the mind as a relaxed alertness and clarity, a general sense of well-being. As one woman succinctly described it: "That walk gets me into a special zone that sets my day."

The enhancement of body-mind well-being as a result of exercise has been linked to the body's secretion of substances called endorphins. These peptides and other circulating messengers, or neurotransmitters, travel through the body and bind to cell receptors, and induce changes in cell metabolism. Neuropharmacologist Candace Pert has called endorphins "biochemical units of emotion" because their activity fluctuates with varying emotions.

Physical activity provides several specific benefits for women:

Reduced stress. Paul Dudley White, dean of American cardiology, termed exercise "the best antidote for nervous and emotional stress." Doing physical activity in the morning allows you to handle more easily the pressures that may arise during the day. Doing it in the evening allows you to release the pressures that accumulate during the day. Numerous studies have shown a clear relationship between regular physical activity on the one hand and stress reduction and increased mental alertness on the other.

I once suggested to Helen, a forty-nine-year-old high-powered businesswoman, that she get away from the stresses at work by taking a walk during the day. She promptly began walking two to three miles daily, and soon was taking her cordless telephone along on her walks. During one office visit, she proudly announced to me, "These days I can walk three miles a day without any problem. In fact, it feels so good that I save the toughest business calls for my walks." Needless to say, I had to tell Helen that this was not exactly what I had in mind.

Improved eating habits and weight control. Physical activity makes it easier for a woman to alter her eating habits comfortably *and* control her weight. Several studies have suggested that exercise leads to changes in the appetite "set point" and improvement in metabolic function—both of which mean easier weight control. Virtually all weight-loss programs now employ exercise as an integral component. This is particularly important for women, since for them excess weight is more of a risk factor for heart disease than it is for men.

Often, simple exercise provides two distinct benefits for the price of one commitment. After starting to exercise regularly on her stationary cycle, for example, an overweight fifty-two-year-old patient told me, "I felt sloppy and sluggish for years. Now I'm thirty pounds lighter—and my mind feels a hundred pounds lighter!"

Reduced blood pressure. Studies indicate that regular exercise lowers the blood pressure of hypertensive patients—

often dramatically, in overweight women with hypertension. Many overweight women have been able to lessen or even eliminate their medication for high blood pressure after they start exercising regularly. The combination of exercise and weight control, besides causing a substantial reduction in blood pressure and heart disease risk, can improve the performance of the heart.

Increased HDL cholesterol and decreased triglyceride levels. Exercise is an excellent way to boost a woman's all-important good (HDL) cholesterol. By so doing, it improves the ratio between total cholesterol and good cholesterol. Exercise also lowers the level of triglycerides, blood lipids that may contribute to the risk of heart disease more in women than in men (see chapter 5).

Improved heart function. Physical activity conditions the heart muscle, making it stronger and more efficient. A conditioned heart beats more slowly at rest, and its rate does not increase as much with exercise. Its pumping action is more efficient because the resistance of blood vessels decreases; when they are more relaxed and open, the heart does not have to work as hard. Aerobic (rhythmic) exercise is the best means of obtaining these benefits to the cardiovascular system. Isometric (sustained, static) exercise builds and contours muscles but does not result in cardiovascular fitness. Walking, hiking, jogging, and swimming are aerobic exercises, while weightlifting is an example of isometric exercise.

TAKING ACTION

Below are suggestions for some activities for you to begin an exercise program. Choose an activity that you will

enjoy. You may want to make your exercise a social opportunity. Try walking, cycling, or doing aerobics with a friend
or family member. The company may reinforce your commitment. If exercise is new for you, begin slowly, with a
mild one. Keep in mind, of course, that there are other
activities for you to engage in.

Walking. This is a favorite for many women because it
is easy and convenient. You can start by just going for a
15-minute walk. Move at your own pace three times a week
for two weeks; increase the time to 20 minutes after the
second walk and to 30 minutes after the first week. By week
three, you can move up from three to four times a week. As
you become more accustomed to walking, and more fit,
increase your pace by lengthening your stride. Most
women can stroll a mile in 30 minutes. Within two to three
weeks, you can become comfortable walking a mile in 20
minutes. To warm up, stroll for the first 3 minutes before
advancing to the desired pace. On days when you feel more
energy, quicken your pace, swing your arms, breathe
deeply, and let go. If you have the chance, walk in the
woods or on the beach. In inclement weather, try a walk in
a shopping mall or another protected location.

Swimming. This wonderfully relaxing exercise allows
you to work your upper and lower muscle groups, while
gliding comfortably through the water. It is particularly
good for women with physical injuries, since it is not a
weight-bearing exercise and does not stress the back or the
joints. Related activities—pool walking, pool jogging, and
pool aerobics have all become popular and provide a nice
workout.

Find a pool you like (preferably heated) and swim laps

at an easy pace. Vary your stroke if you like: freestyle, backstroke, breaststroke, sidestroke, and so on. Begin with a 15-minute swim three times a week for the first week; increase to 20 minutes the second week, and 30 minutes the third week. Pause between laps if you feel tired. By week four, you can swim four times a week.

Cycling. The most important factor in successful cycling is having the right bike: one that rides well and is stable and comfortable. Begin with a casual 15-minute ride on a flat path, setting the gears so that pedaling is easy. Progress comfortably from three 15-minute rides the first week to three 20-minute rides the second week, to three 30-minute rides the third week. By the end of week four, you can go 30 minutes four times a week. To avoid overdoing it, use the "talk test": you should be able to carry on a conversation without difficulty, not needing to time your words with your breathing. If you can't talk comfortably, slow down!

Indoor options. You have many choices if you prefer to exercise indoors. There are stationary bikes, treadmills, rowing machines, stepping machines, and cross-country skiing simulators, among other hardware. Aerobics is a popular choice; whether you take a class or follow an aerobics video, go with a style and a tempo that feel right. If you're exercising at home, find a location that appeals to you, where you can watch television or video, listen to music, read, or do whatever else you like while you work out.

Some of you might want to join a health club. The group energy there attracts many women, as does the variety of indoor machines available. And classes in aerobics, aerobic dance, free weights, and so on can offer a great workout—and be a lot of fun.

FOR THE "COUCH POTATO"

For those of you who have been sedentary most of your lives, the good news is that you have the most to gain from even the simplest physical activities. Gradually work them into your daily life. Start with small, comfortable activities, for instance:

- Walking to your destination whenever it is feasible.
- Taking stairs now and then instead of relying exclusively on elevators.
- Doing more physical tasks around the house or yard.
- Strolling around the block, around your neighborhood, in the park, at the mall.

You may want to develop a support system by having a friend or family member come along. Keep your activity comfortable, and keep it easy. Above all, keep it a part of your life.

POTENTIAL PITFALLS

Although more women are exercising now than ever before, some women still have an aversion to physical activity. Underlying this aversion are feelings of self-defeat, yet women will give any of a number of reasons for not exercising. Among the most common of these pitfalls of rationalization:

1. "I'm not the athletic type," or "I have never exercised, not even as a child." Just remember that you don't have to be a world-class athlete to take a walk. By maintaining a regular program—be it walking or cycling or swimming or aerobics or whatever—you can be healthier, and feel how rewarding good health is. When you are starting a program, however, avoid being pressured into attempting too much by a zealous partner.

2. "I have too much to do to exercise." Many women, it is true, have limited time, and seem always to be doing things for others rather than for themselves. Physical activity is something you are entitled to, for yourself. Remember that this means an expenditure of only a half-hour three or four times a week. The best way to make physical activity a priority is to make *yourself* a priority.

Many women today have overcrowded schedules that seem impossible to change, particularly for something that may appear unimportant, as exercise does to some. With all the other activities women are committed to, physical activity may not be a priority. To avoid this neglect of your body, make your physical activity program a high priority at least for the first four to six weeks. After that, your program should have become a regular part of your life.

Give some thought to what time of day would be best for you. For some women, exercise is an invigorating way to start the day; for others, an evening activity provides a good release to the pressures of the day; to yet others, a midday exercise break feels right. Try out various times of day, and even combinations, but be realistic. If, for example, you already have a full early morning, with meetings to attend or children to get off to school, or if you are not a morning person, exercise in the evening or at midday. Exercise should be *your* time to take control and do something for yourself.

After you have decided the best time, schedule it: write it into your date book or calendar, just as you would any other important appointment. Since you are scheduling this activity for only a half-hour three or four times a week, you have plenty of flexibility. Keep in mind that weekends are a great time to exercise.

3. "I'm too tired to exercise." If excessive demands are made on you as they are on many women, you may feel tired the entire day. Naturally, when you're exhausted, the last thing you feel like doing is exercising; you are assuming that physical activity will use the little energy you have left. In fact, what most women experience after moderate physical activity is a feeling of having more energy, of being more alert, because of the release of those endorphins. Moderate physical activity does not enervate—it invigorates. Try it and see for yourself, as a patient of mine did.

Jill's story is a perfect example. I remember how upset she was when she came to see me several years ago; because she was so exhausted by the stresses of her job and housework that she would fall asleep soon after dinner every night. We discussed exercise, and somewhat reluctantly, she began taking a twenty-minute walk after work. Now, after work Jill goes to an aerobics class. Afterward she feels relaxed, not worn out, and she can enjoy the evening with her family.

4. "Exercise is boring" and "I have more important things to do." Although physical activity may *look* boring, it does not have to *be* boring. I often find that new, interesting thoughts, and solutions to problems, pop into my mind while I walk.

The time spent doing physical activity is hardly

wasted, and it can even do double duty. Ann, a sixty-two-year-old businesswoman I know, takes lunchtime walks twice a week with her business partner. They have found this a useful way to discuss overall goals, long-range planning, and other business matters. In addition, they have gotten to know each other better and have become closer.

There are plenty of other specific—and simple—ways to avoid boredom during physical activity:

If you walk or bike outdoors take along a small radio or a Walkman. If you exercise indoors, turn on the radio, stereo, or CD or cassette player. Try a variety of sounds: quiet music can be relaxing, faster music invigorating, conversation and book or lecture tapes more challenging. If you are outdoors, pay attention to your surroundings, especially in heavy traffic or congested areas.

Exercise with a friend or family member. Having a partner can help you keep your commitment, and may provide other benefits as well. Sheila was a seventy-two-year-old retired schoolteacher who always would be accompanied by her husband when she came for an office visit. Each visit was a repeat of the previous one. Sheila would pull out a long list of the same questions she had asked me on the last visit, and she and her husband would argue over her answers to my questions about how she was doing. As time passed, however, I noticed a difference. Sheila's list grew shorter and shorter, then disappeared. The squabbling between Sheila and her husband decreased, and they actually became sweet with each other. One day I told them, "You really have changed since you first started coming here." "Yes," Sheila said, "now that we've been taking long walks together along the Schuylkill every other day!"

You can make this a special time. Notice the scenery

and the people around you. Vary the route, vary your pace, breathe deeply and relax into your exercise. This is a gift to yourself; if you feel you are being self-indulgent or irresponsible cramming exercise into an already crowded day, remember that you deserve this opportunity.

5. "I don't like to sweat." Some women feel that sweating is uncomfortable or unfeminine. Sweating is a physical release—of all those frustrations and stresses that build up in everyone. It is a healthy outlet for pent-up feelings—especially when compared with smoking, drinking, or eating, which are unhealthy ways of suppressing those feelings. Of course, if sweating is really uncomfortable for you, the best exercise may be swimming.

GETTING STARTED

Write specific, concrete answers to the following:

1. What is my exercise goal for the next month?

2. After choosing an activity from the "Taking Action" section, or another exercise, how will I start?

3. When will I start? If not right now, on what day?

4. How will I stick with my plan? What strategies will I use to keep going?

5. What pitfalls may get in my way?

6. What will I do to handle these pitfalls, or avoid them altogether?

RECORDING YOUR PROGRESS

Enter the following information in a notebook:

Date

How much did I exercise? How far did I go? How much time
did I invest?

Did any pitfalls come up?

What can I learn from today?

IF YOU WANT TO GO FURTHER

Some of you may wish to engage in more strenuous
physical activity such as jogging, cycling faster and far-
ther, or doing high-intensity aerobics. Before beginning
this type of program, check with your physician if you are
past menopause and/or have other heart disease risk factors or if you have a heart disorder. A stress test may be
recommended to detect possible heart problems and to
establish your fitness level.

You can monitor a vigorous workout by determining
your heart rate and, even more basically, seeing how you
feel. To find out your heart rate, position the tips of your
index and middle fingers just below the thumb "fat pad,"
between the wrist bone and tendon. Pressing lightly, feel
and count your pulse for 15 seconds; multiply by 4 to get
your pulse rate per minute. On the basis of your heart rate
and general condition, your physician will be able to provide an "exercise prescription." The principle, as always,
is to start slowly and proceed gradually.

If you want to jog, I suggest you begin with 30 minutes of brisk walking four times a week for two weeks, with a target heart rate 50 percent more than (or one and a half times) your resting rate. If your resting pulse rate is 80 beats per minute, for instance, walk at a pace at which the rate increases to 120 beats per minute. When you are able to walk two miles comfortably in 30 minutes, alternate the brisk walk with a slow jog, allowing 10 minutes for the jog and 20 minutes for the walk. During the jog, allow your pulse rate to increase to 60 to 70 percent higher than your resting rate. When this becomes comfortable, phase into 15 minutes of jogging and 15 minutes of brisk walking, then to 20 of jogging and 10 of brisk walking, and finally to 30 minutes of jogging three or four times a week.

I recommend keeping your pulse rate while jogging at 70 percent of your maximal heart rate. While some authorities allow for as much as 85 percent, the lower percentage is sensible because it gives you a solid training effect with less stress on the heart. To determine your target heart rate, subtract your age from 220 and take 70 percent of this number. If you are sixty years old, for example, your target rate is 112: 220 minus 60 is 160, and 70 percent of 160 is 112.

Keep in mind two safety factors: First, warm up (before) and cool down (after) with at least 10 minutes of stretching, and start your jog slowly. Second, pay attention to your body and how you feel. Go at a comfortable pace, and if you do not feel well, stop. Chest discomfort or pressure, severe shortness of breath, irregular heartbeat, nausea, excessive fatigue, or dizziness are all reasons to stop and consult your physician. While jogging, use the "talk test": If you cannot carry on a conversation easily, slow down. Even more strenuous physical activity should feel comfortable.

TO SUM UP

1. Physical activity is the most direct and effective way for a woman to discover the wonder of her body. It is the best first step to health.

2. The equivalent of walking thirty minutes a day four times a week provides major health benefits for women.

3. Just as there is a mind-body relationship, through which the body receives messages from the mind, there is a body-mind relationship, whereby the body communicates its messages to the mind. Both mind and body influence each other, in positive or negative ways.

4. When a woman feels bodily discomfort, her blood vessels tend to become constricted and the flow of blood more sluggish. Exercise relaxes the body and opens up the arteries, through the release of endorphins and other neurotransmitters.

5. The benefits of physical activity on the body-mind cycle are seen in several areas: reduced stress, improved eating habits and weight control, reduced blood pressure, increased good cholesterol and decreased triglyceride levels, and improved heart performance.

6. When choosing an exercise program, pick an activity that feels right for you. Make this activity a high priority for at least the first four to six weeks; determine the best time to exercise, enter your plans in your appointment book, and keep this date with yourself. The best way to make physical activity a priority is to make yourself a priority.

7. Whatever activity you select, begin slowly, proceed gradually, and keep things fresh; experiment, and use exercise as a social activity if you like. You will discover that exercise can be a source of energy in your life.

CHAPTER 4

Handling Stress: The Problems Around Us and the Thoughts Within Us

We see things not as they are, but as we are.
What we are, the world is.
KRISHNAMURTI

Today we can have a solid foundation on
which to create and build a life based upon
truth, choice and freedom.
JOYCE SUTTILL

Stress—everyone talks about it, and the national statistics are frightening. It is estimated that 75 percent of all medical complaints are stress-related. Approximately $15 billion are lost by industry annually because of stress-related absenteeism. About 5 billion doses of tranquilizers are prescribed each year. It has long been believed that stress might contribute to heart disease. Until recently this notion has been supported only by anecdotes: the wife who never had a heart problem, but suffered a heart attack soon after the death of her husband; the surge in heart attacks after such traumatic experiences as earthquakes or personal crises. But several medical studies conducted in countries around the world, including the United States, Israel, and Sweden, have provided evidence that emotional stress precedes the onset of symptoms of heart disease, in women as well as men.

What is stress? This question crystallized for me one day when two of my patients, both women, individually asked me the same question: How were their highly demanding jobs affecting their health? I responded with my own question to each of them: "How do you feel about your job?" The first said, "I hate it! I can't stand the environment or the people. And my work bores me." The second answered, "I really like what I do. The atmosphere in the office is exciting, and the work is challenging. Of course, there are times when I'd rather be elsewhere, but you can't expect everything to be perfect." Needless to say, their jobs were affecting the health of these two women very differently. The first had job stress, while the second had job satisfaction. What fascinated me was that these two women were partners in the same business.

As the example above illustrates, stress is not just "out there"; it is not simply a result of circumstances. Stress depends also on how you interpret circumstances, on what your own thoughts and feelings tell you about the circumstances. If you look at stress from this perspective, you have more possibilities for dealing with it. You need no longer be limited to being a victim of circumstance and letting a particular situation control your emotions. It is worthwhile to evaluate your situation, but if you understand your thoughts and feelings about it, you can discover sensible approaches to handling specific problems.

What causes you to view a circumstance as stressful?

Generally, stress is triggered by any situation or event which might appear to control, limit, or undermine your power. Frustration and anger develop when you sense that you are not getting what you want or deserve.

Women tend to become upset when they feel powerless or helpless, unable to change their circumstances. Recent research has shown that hostility in women increases their risk for heart disease and heart attack. The Framingham Heart Study demonstrated not only that high levels of hostility in women increase their risk of heart attack, but also that women married to overly demanding men have an increased risk. Many women feel it is unacceptable to express their feelings in such marriages, and their stress levels increase accordingly.

Such emotions as anger and hostility, translated into stress and turned inward, have significant consequences on the body. Stress brings with it a sense of resistance and diminishment, of contraction and closing down; if you are under stress, you may feel constricted, stuck, irritable. This is precisely how stress is communicated to and by your body, especially your cardiovascular system:

• There is resistance in the coronary arteries, and the flow of blood to the heart diminishes.

• Other blood vessels become contracted, and thereby increase blood pressure.

• The coronary arteries can become more closed down and constricted, and even go into spasm.

• Substances circulating in the blood cause blood platelet elements to develop an increased tendency to get stuck, and thus increase the possibility of blood clots.

• The irritability of the heart increases, and can lead to serious rhythm disturbances.

It is no surprise that anger and hostility play such a significant role in deciding risk of heart disease. At the University of Florida Preventive Cardiology Clinic, an assessment was made of the psychological factors underlying heart disease in 75 men and 41 women. According to Dr. Nancy Norvell, who supervised the study, hostility and anger correlated strongly with increased risk of heart disease.

HOW TO KEEP YOUR PERSPECTIVE AND COPE

Many people tend to become stressed by anticipating or being obsessed with situations over which they have no control. Almost always this involves some level of distorted reality.

Whenever such stress-provoking thoughts come up, ask yourself these questions:

- What is the worst thing that can happen?
- Even if the worst happens, how important will it be to me a year from now? Five years from now?
- If a friend came to me with this situation, what advice would I offer?
- How can I change my distorted thoughts and approach the situation more objectively?

Tell yourself:

- If I look at my track record, one way or another I have *always* managed to come through. I will be okay!

If you are in the midst of a stress reaction, *stop* (go to another room if necessary to disengage from the situation) and take one or two minutes to relax. Use this breathing technique:

Take five slow, deep breaths. For each, inhale to a count of 4, pause for a second, and exhale to a count of 4. As you inhale, visualize a soothing blue vapor filling your body; as you exhale, visualize red-hot tension leaving your body. To help yourself relax, picture a calm natural scene, the seashore or mountains, for example; imagine its beauty and serenity. When you feel sufficiently wound down, ask yourself the reality-based questions listed above.

Studies by Dr. John Barefoot confirm how dangerous the emotion of hostility is to the heart. "People who score high on the hostility scale tend to have a poor risk profile," according to Barefoot. "Conversely, low hostility indicates a lower risk of coronary heart disease."

A study conducted among workers at a Volvo factory in Sweden showed that men and women had the same blood pressure and stress-related hormone responses at the workplace. When the workers went home, the men's blood pressure and stress hormone levels fell, while the women's blood pressure and stress hormone levels remained high. This study gives new meaning to the old axiom that a woman's work is never done.

And yet, there are remedies for stress. Spouses and children can assist in household chores to relieve women of some of their burdens. Children can have specific assignments and clean up after themselves, although this may require firm persistence for a while. Husbands or partners can help with shopping or other specific tasks.

You might do what I often suggest to my female patients who are under stress at home: hold a family meeting at which you discuss the domestic situation with the rest of the household. Before the meeting, sit down and think carefully about the specific changes you want. Write down whatever is necessary or important in reducing your stressful circumstances. Writing things down will help you express yourself fully and bring about meaningful change. Men, as well as children, respond best to concrete, specific, positive statements and requests. You have every right to make these requests, and stating them in a straightforward, unequivocal way may facilitate the results you want.

By now the effects of stress on the cardiovascular system are considered predictable, so much so that mental stress tests are used routinely in many cardiology laboratories to detect heart abnormalities. It is clear that since the mind and the body communicate, stress can lead to serious illness. Not only does stress make the body more vulnerable to illness, but the body may attempt to "resolve" stress through illness.

Linda found this out firsthand. Now a highly successful businesswoman, she worked seven-day weeks for years to build her business and bring up her two children (she is divorced). Although her business was thriving, Linda felt overwhelmed and powerless. How could she slow down, spend time with her kids, *and* maintain the business she already had devoted so much energy to? How could she change the status quo? Her answer came in the form of severe, incapacitating chest pains and shortness of breath. Fortunately, Linda's symptoms were a false alarm and not a heart attack. A medical evaluation revealed no coronary artery disease, and the disorder was diagnosed as mitral valve prolapse, a generally benign condition (described further in chapter 9). Yet the chest pains and difficult breathing provided an excuse for Linda. She was "forced" to get some desperately needed rest and restoration.

It is not just women whose bodies attempt to resolve stress through illness. In 1985, I had a bout with a major illness: a rare allergic reaction to an influenza virus. I just had been appointed chairman of the department of medicine at the hospital where I was already working overtime as director of a heart institute and caring for a large cardiology practice. With the added responsibility, I felt overwhelmed, out of control, and very stressed. My body gave me the perfect solution: First, "it" got the flu and I was forced to bed for five days. When I dragged myself back to work prematurely, my body had an allergic reaction to the bug. Immediately I was back in bed and away from all my responsibilities for a month.

RECOGNIZING STRESS

Certain circumstances inevitably may bring about stress. The most important universal stress triggers for women include death of a relative or close friend, divorce or separation, personal or family illness, difficulty with children, job crisis, sexual difficulty, and financial difficulty. In addition, certain symptoms are important clues to recognizing stress. Among these are unusual fatigue; insomnia; headaches; inability to concentrate or perform tasks; increased use of food, drugs, or alcohol; and illness. You almost certainly are experiencing stress if you are facing a universal stress trigger or experiencing stress-related symptoms.

In addition to the universal triggers, every woman has her own unique factors that cause stress. The first step to handling stress is recognizing specific sources of stress, including negative, hostile, or angry thoughts. A simple exercise may help you identify your personal stress triggers. Take 10 to 15 minutes to write your responses to the following:

1. Circumstances that make me angry are:

2. Circumstances that make me frustrated are:

3. Circumstances that make me hostile are:

4. Circumstances that make me feel powerless are:

5. Circumstances that make me feel a loss of control are:

6. Circumstances that currently are causing the most stress in my life are:

Edna St. Vincent Millay once said, "It is not true that life is one damn thing after another—it's one damn thing over and over." You may believe likewise when you look over your responses. Do you detect any recurring themes or patterns in the circumstances that trigger your reactions? Select the three or four specific circumstances that you would most like to modify. On a sheet of paper, draw a vertical line down the center and write these circumstances on the left. On the right, list corresponding possibilities that would be less stress-provoking.

A personal example: Since I moved to Los Angeles, I have found that driving on the crowded freeways makes me angry, frustrated, hostile, feeling powerless, and so on. One day I was fuming about traffic while driving with my son, Steve. He made a simple suggestion: "Dad, getting uptight isn't going to change anything, so why not sit back, turn on some music, and just relax. We'll get there in the same time, and you'll feel a lot better." I have taken his advice and not only has driving felt easier, but for some strange reason, the traffic doesn't seem so bad—except when I slip. If I were doing the exercise above, on the left side of the paper I would write: "Driving in heavy traffic," and on the right: "Sitting back, turning on music, relaxing."

TAKING ACTION

Recognizing your recurring stress trigger thoughts and beliefs is an important first step. However, the key is believing that it is within your ability to control stress rather than have stress control you. In addition, it is good to remember that taking care of your own needs is the all-important core factor to your being a healthy woman. This four-step approach has worked for women in my practice and for me. It can work for you too.

1. Physical Activity

Exercise is a valuable way to release stress. However, during periods of severe stress we usually feel worn down and unable to exercise—we just want to collapse! Our minds are worn out, but our bodies are tense and constricted. Exercising anyway, regardless of how you feel about it, can be remarkably refreshing and invigorating. Your body and your blood vessels open up, endorphins are released, and a reawakened sense of well-being occurs.

TYPE A BEHAVIOR

Type A behavior was described for the first time in 1959, by Dr. Meyer Friedman, who termed it a medical disorder. Type A behavior is characterized by impatience, free-floating hostility and aggressiveness, easily aroused irritation or anger, high levels of ambition and competitiveness, and a constant sense of urgency. Dr. Friedman also identified people with type B behavior, who are more passive, showing less responsiveness to stress and little sense of urgency. Significantly, he found the premature onset of heart disease seven times more common in type A than in type B individuals.

Since Dr. Friedman's original research, the importance of type A behavior as a risk factor for heart disease has been challenged. More recent studies have not proved a relationship between type A behavior and heart disease. They show instead that states of severe stress, hostility, and anger are more related to cardiovascular risk than is type A behavior per se. My experience with patients has been that those with certain type A characteristics (drive, competitiveness, sense of urgency) who feel productive and good about what they do and who enjoy the challenge of their work are if anything at lower risk than those with type B characteristics who also exhibit evidence of chronic depression.

2. Relaxation Techniques

Learning and using techniques to relax can change your life. Studies have demonstrated that they do promote health. Dr. Herbert Benson, a friend of mine at Harvard, has taken the mystique out of these methods with his pioneering studies showing that proper relaxation, in addition to creating a sense of well-being, can lower blood pressure and even help maintain a normal cholesterol level. I have followed Dr. Benson's work closely, including his book *The Relaxation Response*, yet I started using relaxation methods only because of an unusual experience with a particularly troublesome patient.

Marlene was an obese middle-aged woman with a mild heart problem. Despite repeated assurances that she was stable, Marlene was ridden with fear and anxiety. She called me daily to talk about her "terrible condition," and several nights a week the emergency room would inform me that Marlene was back with another false alarm. Suddenly, however, this pattern stopped: no more phone calls from Marlene, no emergency room visits. About six months later, when she appeared in my office waiting room, I barely recognized her. It was not just that she had lost a lot of weight; there was something else very different about her. "I don't need to see you," she told me, and this obviously was true—"but I've discovered something that has changed my life and that could really help *you*." "Oh, really? And what is that?" I asked in disbelief. "I meditate," she answered quietly. Marlene was right about my needing help. At the time, I was very stressed, and willing to try anything. I went back to Dr. Benson's book and started practicing relaxation techniques. I have been grateful to Marlene ever since.

Aside from its specific health benefits, the "relaxation response" offers a practical and effective way to gain a new perspective on the thoughts and feelings that often trigger stress. The insights possible with this uniquely calm state of mind can help defuse stress triggers and the stress itself. It also is a process whereby you can reevaluate your thoughts naturally and spontaneously.

The relaxation method is simple:

• Find a quiet place, with surroundings that are comfortable, where you will not be disturbed.

• Sit on a chair or on the floor, quietly and in a comfortable upright position.

• Pick a word or phrase to concentrate on. This can be a word, such as "peace," "love," or "trust"; a pleasing sound; or a phrase or sentence, such as "I choose to live today in peace"—whatever feels comfortable and right to you. Or gaze at an object or picture that is meaningful. Or simply concentrate your attention on your breath as it goes slowly and deeply in and out.

• Assume a passive attitude. Above all, do not worry about how you are doing. When intrusive thoughts come into your mind, simply say to yourself, "Aha" or "Interesting," let them go, and return to your focus.

It is recommended that you relax in this manner for 10 to 20 minutes once or twice a day. I have found that even as little as 5 to 10 minutes in the morning is beneficial, although 10 minutes is preferable. According to Dr. Benson, the two essential elements are the repetition of the word or sound and the passive attitude to release intrusive thoughts.

Relaxing, or meditating, may require some effort on

two fronts. You need to make a commitment to do it, first of all, and then ignore doubts about how you are doing. When I began meditating, a voice inside me would say things like, "This feels strange. Do you really want to do this?" and "You're doing this all wrong. This isn't it," and "Forget it. You'll never get it right." Be aware that you may have this initial doubt. To have a realistic chance for the relaxation response to take hold, commit to meditating daily for three weeks—no matter what the commentator in your mind says. A feeling for it will evolve slowly over the three weeks, and potentially distracting thoughts remain just thoughts rather than judgments. When they are not as pervasive or forceful, you will be able to focus and will begin to feel the benefits of the relaxation response.

The value of relaxation is profound for both peace of mind and performance. The only trick is to do it. After a morning relaxation exercise, you will enjoy a sense of calmness and alertness. You will feel refreshed and more in control, and protected from the possibly trying circumstances of the day ahead. Things that ordinarily upset you no longer have that effect: they are more interesting than irritating, or you are less reactive and more detached toward them. You see more objectively and are more effective in handling yourself and your situation.

VISUALIZATION

Visualizing is a wonderful way to relax during the morning or to offset a stressful event during the day. Close your eyes and imagine a time and a place in which you were completely at peace. It might have been at the seashore, in the mountains, near a stream in the woods, or in a cozy den, in front of a warm fire. Capture the scene vividly, in detail, using as many of your senses as you can: see the wide sky or the play of sun and shade, smell the fresh air or homey scents, listen to the gurgling or splashing water. Feel the tranquility of the scene inside yourself. You can return to this special place as often as you like, to find the inner serenity needed to start your day or restore a balanced perspective when you are upset. Even a few moments in your imaginary time and place can have lasting benefits.

3. Written Communication

Writing about your thoughts and the events in your life is a productive way to get at what is really happening under the surface. When you put your important concerns and your feelings about them down on paper, they become crystallized and clarified. They can be seen more objectively. Putting your concerns on paper also seems to place boundaries around them: they no longer appear all-encompassing or overwhelming. Writing them down in front of you makes them less vague, more visible, more manageable.

NEWS OF THE WEEK

When you record specific events, even in as brief a session as 15 minutes a week, you develop a sort of control over them. It is you who collects them, chooses the more significant ones, and then puts them into words. This sense of control about your own news of the week helps you understand the core of things. Solutions seem to come spontaneously from another, wiser part of you.

Write about what is happening, for instance the circumstances that are causing stress; about how you feel and think about these circumstances; and about how you can change your approach to them. But your news may not be all stress-related. Write also about your positive news, and how you might use it to counter any stressful events.

LETTER WRITING

Writing a letter—but *not* sending it—to someone with whom you have stressful problems may help you understand the situation better and perhaps resolve it. You can write such a letter to your boss, coworkers, husband, children, other relatives—and even yourself. Express exactly how and why you are upset and what you think about the person when you are upset. State what you really want in the troublesome situation, and in the relationship in general. Understand that the purpose of such a letter is strictly personal, for *you* to gain insight and resolve conflicts.

You also can try the reverse—an imaginary letter to you from the person with whom you are having problems. This enterprise may seem strange, but it can give you a new understanding of another individual. You can appreciate what might be motivating the person's behavior and can, accordingly, modify your reactions to that behavior. This can be helpful in solving personal problems.

REEVALUATING YOUR OWN STRESS TRIGGERS

The written exercise in the "Recognizing Stress" section can provide ongoing insights into your thinking patterns. Since our beliefs determine how we interpret and react to circumstances, some of them are well worth reevaluating. Research at the University of Pennsylvania, among other institutions, has shown that the recurrent thoughts that cause stress, even though they may appear reasonable and right, nearly always contain distortions. Do the stress recognition exercise regularly, to recall which distorted beliefs continue to trigger stress. Then see if you can let such beliefs go.

4. Spoken Communication

Just as writing allows you to "read" yourself, others, and stressful situations more objectively, speaking allows you to hear yourself more objectively. When you "think out loud," you may receive valuable feedback from an external source. Communicating feelings aloud requires trust; in this respect women are more trusting than men, much better at expressing their feelings. Men tend to hold back because they are afraid of being vulnerable, of not looking good, of being misunderstood, or worst of all, of being rejected. In addition, male conditioning has been to keep a stiff upper lip. We all, women as well as men, need to remember that in times of severe stress, our hearts are psychologically and physically "under attack." If you are uncomfortable talking intimately with a friend, or if doing so does not seem to be adequate, professional help or a support group may be worthwhile. Certainly, if you are under severe stress, the advice of a professional counselor is invaluable.

Vulnerability is after all a human trait, everyone experiences it at some time. When stress becomes overwhelming and you feel out of control, you are entitled to acknowledge it and find support. Being under great stress is painful, but if you get the proper assistance, it can also become a unique opportunity to learn, to grow, to understand and change long-standing feelings or habits that have not been serving you. Working through your stress can become a powerful way to heal your heart physically, emotionally, and spiritually.

A POTENTIAL PITFALL

As I have stated before, it is not just specific circumstances themselves that cause stress, but also certain self-defeating thoughts, feelings, and interpretations. You must be willing to acknowledge and tend to your own needs if you are to break the cycle of stress in your life, to obtain meaningful benefits from this chapter. Negative thoughts— "This isn't for me," or "I don't really need this," or "I don't have time for this"—are barriers to change. You can try to be stoic, but while you fight to keep up a strong front, the stress can affect your body and your health. In fact, spasm of the coronary arteries has been linked directly to stress. Severe stress, then, may set you up for a heart attack.

If however, your thoughts are open and positive— "I'm going to try this, I'm worth it," or "What do I have to lose?"—you will feel engaged and energized. These thoughts can open up your mind and your body, including your blood vessels. This optimistic attitude also will open realistic opportunities to make your life less stressful and give you a sense of control.

You *can* avoid the pitfall of negative thinking to invalidate the possibility for change. It may seem to you that your problems are too difficult or not even important enough to deal with and resolve. The material in this chapter can work for you, if you work with it. It can provide you with a sense of control and effectiveness, as well as a more quiet, peaceful mind and heart.

GETTING STARTED

Write specific, concrete answers to the following:

1. What is my goal to handle and reduce stress for the next month? What specific area of stress do I choose to deal with?

2. After choosing methods of handling stress from the "Taking Action" section, how will I start?

3. When will I start? If not right now, on what day?

4. How will I stick with my plan? What techniques will I use to keep going?

5. What pitfalls may get in my way?

6. What will I do to handle these pitfalls, or avoid them altogether?

RECORDING YOUR PROGRESS

Enter the following information in a notebook:

Date

What universal stress triggers came up today, and what
were the circumstances?

What was my own stress trigger?

Am I using physical activity, relaxation, writing, and spoken communication to control stress, and did I employ
them today?

Did any pitfalls come up?

What can I learn from today?

TO SUM UP

1. Medical studies from around the world have shown
that stress frequently precedes symptoms of heart disease.

2. Stress is not due simply to external circumstances.
It results largely from what your thoughts tell you about a
situation, how your mind interprets it.

3. Stress arises whenever your thoughts interpret a
specific circumstance as a threat—something that you think
will control or limit you, or take away your power to obtain
what you want or think you deserve.

4. Stress is communicated directly to the body, particularly the cardiovascular system, by constriction of the
coronary arteries; contraction of other blood vessels, and
consequent high blood pressure; increased possibility of
blood clots; and heart rhythm disturbances. Not only does
stress make the body more vulnerable to illness, but the

body may attempt to resolve and relieve stress through illness.

5. You *can* control stress; my recommended approach to understanding and handling it includes physical activity, even though you might think you're too exhausted; relaxation techniques, even though they may seem strange initially; written communication, even though your reports and letters don't leave your hands; and spoken communication, even though it may seem indulgent.

6. Negative thinking can weaken your attempts to manage stress. Using this program with a positive, open attitude is the key to a calm, effective, *healthy* life.

CHAPTER 5

Healthy Eating: Being Well Fed, Not Fed Up

You may have to fight a battle more than once to win it.
MARGARET THATCHER

One swallow does not a summer make.
ARISTOTLE

"FED UP!" read a recent cover of *Newsweek*, which went on to ask, "Is There Anything Left We Can Eat?" No area of health has been more confusing and misunderstood than diet and nutrition, especially as related to cholesterol levels and the risk of heart disease. Many women today think that eating properly means cutting out everything they love, and thus feeling deprived and dissatisfied. I remember one of my patients bringing in a magazine article about nutrition that she wanted to discuss. As she showed it to me, she said, "You doctors make it sound like we have to live on sprouts, oat bran, and tofu, while I walk around hungry and miserable all day!''

The facts are that eating healthily and reducing your risk of heart disease do *not* have to involve pain and sacrifice. In all likelihood, many of your favorite foods are healthy, and many of your favorite recipes can be modified easily to become healthy. Proper eating is not difficult and does not have to be complicated; it requires only a few simple adjustments.

Women can learn to eat well and teach others to do likewise by following one rule and keeping one commitment. The rule: Cut down the fat, by making simple substitutions. This decreases not only cholesterol levels but also the number of calories. The commitment: Set aside your preconceived notions about food and become a thoughtful eater. Being a thoughtful eater means thinking clearly and objectively about the food you eat; making adjustments and substitutions more knowledgeably and comfortably; experimenting and learning what works best for you; introducing changes over time rather than abruptly; and allowing for slips. Being a thoughtful eater also means becoming interested in learning relevant information about food and health.

Mary, a feisty saleswoman, was overweight and had high blood pressure and very high total cholesterol and low good cholesterol levels when she first came to see me. She was also a confessed junk-food eater. "I just don't listen to any of that stuff about everything being bad for you," she told me. I responded that her cholesterol, blood pressure, and weight put her at high risk for serious heart problems, but that by learning to eat sensibly she could decrease her risk substantially. She became very quiet, then asked whether I had any written information for her to read. I gave her a few pamphlets provided by the American Heart Association.

Soon Mary was deluging me with articles about nutrition. She had become a self-proclaimed "food connoisseur" and had decided to become my nutrition consultant. Her weight, blood pressure, and cholesterol level eventually came down to normal. Mary discovered that eating well does not have to be drudgery. "Food shopping used to be a bore," she admitted, "but since I learned something about it, I feel like James Bond figuring out those food labels."

HOW TO CALCULATE THE AMOUNT OF FAT YOU MAY EAT

To determine your daily allowable fat intake, first determine your calorie needs. Women require about 13 calories a day per pound of ideal body weight, while men need about 15. Thus, if your ideal weight is 120 pounds, multiply by 13: $120 \times 13 = 1,560$ calories a day. To calculate your total fat calories, multiply your total calories by the fat percentage. If, for example, you have chosen the 30 percent suggested by the American Heart Association, and your daily calorie total is 1,560: $1,560 \times .30 = 468$; you may have 468 calories from fat daily. To determine the actual amount of fat in grams, divide the number of calories by 9 (1 gram of fat provides 9 calories): $468 \div 9 = 52$, so 468 calories of fat corresponds to 52 grams. Now that you know how to figure out your daily fat allowance, you can read food labels more purposefully. For further information, see "How to Decode Food Labels" on page 75.

CHOLESTEROL, TRIGLYCERIDES, AND THE RISK OF HEART DISEASE

All the evidence indicates a direct relationship between high total blood cholesterol levels and the risk of developing coronary heart disease. The National Cholesterol Education Program and the American Heart Association have classified cholesterol levels as follows:

below 200—desirable
200 to 239—borderline high
240 and above—high

Because coronary heart disease is rare in societies in which cholesterol levels are around 150, some experts feel that this level is ideal. A cholesterol level of 250 is associated with twice the coronary heart disease risk of a 200 level, while a cholesterol level of 300 represents four times the risk of a 200 level.

The classifications cited above, it should be noted, are based largely on studies of men. Research suggests that the relationship between total cholesterol and coronary heart disease risk may be different for women. The relative levels of good (high-density lipoprotein, or HDL) and bad (low-density lipoprotein, or LDL) cholesterol appear to be more important than the total cholesterol level alone in determining a woman's risk. Laboratories usually report a ratio between levels of total cholesterol and good cholesterol, with high good cholesterol levels yielding a lower ratio. Current information indicates that a woman is at risk when her ratio exceeds 4.0. If your total cholesterol is 240 and your good cholesterol is 80, your ratio is 3.0. If the same total cholesterol of 240 is accompanied by a good cholesterol of only 40, your ratio would be 6.0 and would represent a risk.

This ratio, then, is all-important, as a recent National Institutes of Health panel agreed. According to that panel, even when total cholesterol is at a desirable level, below 200, there may be significant risk for heart disease if good cholesterol is below 35. And an elevated total cholesterol level of 200 to 240, if accompanied by good cholesterol of 70 or above, is not associated with a significant risk.

Triglyceride levels seem to play a greater role in determining the risk of heart disease for women than for men. It is therefore important that you know this value and keep it under control. Triglyceride levels of 150 to 250 are considered normal by most authorities. Not long ago, however, an international medical panel recommended treatment when the level exceeded 200. One of the reasons for this is the apparent inverse relationship between triglycerides and good cholesterol levels: lowering triglyceride levels has been shown to cause an increase in good cholesterol levels. (See "Cholesterol, Atherosclerosis, and Triglycerides" below.)

CHOLESTEROL, ATHEROSCLEROSIS, AND TRIGLYCERIDES

Cholesterol is a fatlike substance normally used by the body to form cell membranes and certain hormones. It is transported through the bloodstream by special carriers called lipoproteins, the two most important being low-density lipoproteins (LDL) and high-density lipoproteins (HDL).

Too much LDL, or bad cholesterol, increases the risk of cholesterol plaque, a buildup that can clog one of the coronary arteries and lead to heart attack if the artery closes off. This process is known as *atherosclerosis*. Dietary factors are the major cause of high LDL; genetics also plays a role.

HDL, or good cholesterol, is believed to remove cholesterol from the arteries and transport it to the liver. A high level of HDL has been shown to decrease the likelihood of heart attack, while a low level increases the risk. The major reversible causes for low HDL are cigarette smoking, obesity, and lack of exercise.

An LDL level of more than 160 is considered high risk; 130 to 160 borderline high; and less than 130 low risk. An HDL level of less than 35 is an independent risk.

Triglycerides are fat substances whose significance has been controversial; more recent studies indicate that high levels constitute a risk factor for heart disease in women. While most authorities consider desirable triglyceride levels to be below 250, some suggest that they are better kept below 200.

DIETARY FAT AND THE RISK OF HEART DISEASE

The American Heart Association, the National Cholesterol Education Program, and the National Research Council have all recommended that women as well as men obtain no more than 30 percent of their daily total calories from fat, and that they decrease their intake of cholesterol and saturated fat, which increases total cholesterol. Women who have a high percentage of fat in their diet have correspondingly high levels of total cholesterol, bad cholesterol, and triglyceride. A high-fat diet is also a high-calorie diet; there are more calories in fat than in protein or carbohydrates. A gram of fat contains 9 calories, while a gram of protein or carbohydrate contains only 4 calories. This disparity is significant: overweight women are at risk for heart disease.

Two doctors, Dean Ornish and David Blankenhorn, have concluded independently that by reducing total cholesterol levels to about 150–160, atherosclerosis will not develop and, if already present, it will be reversed. Drs. Ornish and Blankenhorn recommend a diet of 10 percent fat (i.e., a vegetarian diet) to achieve these lower cholesterol levels. This is also the diet recommended by the Pritikin program.

IF YOU WANT TO GO FURTHER: THE ORNISH AND PRITIKIN DIETS

Recent research by two independent investigators, Dean Ornish and David Blankenhorn, has suggested that a diet in which 10 percent of daily calories come from fat can prevent, and indeed reverse, coronary artery blockages. This percentage is the same as that long advocated by the Pritikin program. While information on the benefits of diets this low in fat is preliminary—although very promising—and while most authorities have yet to accept the recommendations of these investigators, it is worthwhile to explore and understand such diets.

Low-fat regimes rely primarily on fresh fruits and

vegetables and whole-grain foods. Dr. Ornish's Reversal Diet includes no oils, no animal products except egg whites and nonfat milk and yogurt, and no caffeine or other stimulants or MSG, but it does permit moderate use of salt and sugar. Dr. Ornish's studies have led him to believe that the American Heart Association allowance of 30 percent of total calories from fat is too much to reverse coronary heart disease. Dr. Ornish advocates a prevention diet for people without coronary heart disease, which allows for 20 percent of total calories from fat. (To understand how to interpret the various percentages in terms of actual food, see "How to Calculate the Amount of Fat You May Eat" on page 64.)

If you have the motivation and if a diet with 10 to 20 percent fat can work for you—long-term—by all means go for it. But if that seems too severe, start a diet with 30 percent fat or less. If you then decide to reduce further, you will have a powerful springboard toward success.

An Expert Panel Report issued by the National Cholesterol Education Program in 1991, however, maintains that one need not resort to such low levels of dietary fat, 10 to 20 percent of total calories for example, to reduce blood cholesterol levels, "provided that intakes of saturated fatty acids are kept low." My experience has been that while a vegetarian diet may be a laudable goal, it is not realistic for most people.

My view of the current information is as follows:

A total cholesterol level of below 200 is an important and sensible goal. It is also important, though, to have your cholesterol and triglyceride levels and your total-to-HDL-cholesterol ratio checked regularly. You thereby can understand your risk of heart disease more completely and determine what you need to do specifically to decrease that risk.

If your cholesterol and triglyceride levels are especially high, repeat the tests. They are somewhat difficult to perform accurately, and laboratory errors do occur. Two sets of values from a reputable lab that are in agreement and exceed the recommended values can be trusted, and acted on. Begin by changing your eating habits. Decrease your total fat consumption to 30 percent or less of total calories, your saturated fat intake to less than 10 percent of total calories, and your cholesterol intake to less than 300 milligrams daily. Have your cholesterol and triglyceride levels checked after about six weeks. If they are still not satisfactory, you may want to decrease total fat intake further, to 10 or 20 percent of total calories. Some people at this point may need to consider a cholesterol-lowering drug.

A low level of good cholesterol may be due to cigarette smoking, sedentary life-style, excessive weight, or high sugar intake. If low HDL is your problem, choose the remedy or remedies that apply to you: quit smoking, exercise, lose weight, cut down on sugar, lower your triglyceride level, if it is elevated. Medications to increase HDL are also available; consult your doctor about these.

If your *triglycerides are elevated*, the most efficient ways to decrease them are to reduce your weight, exercise, decrease your sugar intake, and avoid alcohol.

Correcting abnormalities in fat and cholesterol levels does decrease the risk of heart disease in women. There is even evidence that improving these levels may be more effective in preventing atherosclerosis and causing its regression in women than in men.

I have found that the approach that has worked best for women is not "going on a diet," but gradually, thoughtfully, and flexibly altering their eating habits. Diets usually don't last. This was communicated very clearly to me by one of my patients, a fifty-three-year-old politician. She interrupted my "diet talk" by saying, "Please don't tell me how to diet. Tell me how to *eat!*" When you slowly modify how you eat, you will have better long-term results; you can experiment, learn what works and what doesn't, and allow your taste buds and stomach to adjust.

TAKING ACTION

Below are some suggestions for dietary changes. These are meant as general guidelines; you may want to adjust some or make other changes in your own eating plan. Pay close attention to the food you eat, and cut down on fat whenever possible by making simple substitutions. You might want to consult with a registered dietitian or a nutritionist for assistance with specific food choices.

Seven Substitutions

1. Use skim (0.5 percent fat) or low-fat (1 to 2 percent fat) milk and cheese, soft-tub (not stick) margarine, and nonfat yogurt in place of whole milk and regular cheese, butter, and ice cream.

2. Eat more fish and poultry (with skin removed) and complex carbohydrates such as pasta, rice, potatoes, and whole-grain bread. Eat lean cuts of meat, with the fat trimmed away, in smaller (e.g., 4-ounce) portions.

3. Use egg whites and/or egg substitutes instead of egg yolks.

4. Avoid high-cholesterol organ foods such as liver, kidney, brain, sweetbreads.

5. Cut back on processed meats such as sausage, bologna, corned beef, pastrami, salami, and hot dogs. This doesn't mean you have to give up sandwiches; try chicken or turkey breast, with margarine and mustard instead of butter and mayo.

6. Adopt healthier methods of cooking: boil, steam, broil, roast, or bake instead of frying.

7. Choose salad dressings and sauces made with unsaturated oils (corn, canola, safflower, soybean, cottonseed, sunflower, olive), and avoid saturated oils (coconut, palm, palm kernel). Flavor your meals with herbs and seasonings instead of butter and fatty sauces.

A reasonable goal would be to cut down on red meat and processed meat, whole-milk products, and egg yolks, to a maximum of twice a week each for one or two weeks, and to once a week after that. There are many flexible alternatives to accommodate your individual tastes. If you like cheese, eat that instead of red meat; perhaps substitute a skim-milk cheese, such as mozzarella or ricotta, or low-fat cottage cheese. If cutting down on red meat is too hard, have it lean, trimmed of fat and in smaller portions. Make scrambled eggs or omelets with one egg yolk and extra egg white; use any of the various egg substitutes available. If you have a sweet tooth, select low-fat baked goods made with unsaturated oils and unfrosted cakes and cookies in place of gooey, rich desserts, and switch from ice cream to nonfat frozen yogurt or a nonfat frozen dessert.

A sixty-five-year-old celebrity patient of mine, who was overweight and had a significantly elevated cholesterol level, claimed to be hooked on a well-known brand of ice cream. "Have you ever tried nonfat frozen yogurt?" I asked. "My daughter, Sharon, introduced me to it several years ago and we've both become hooked on *it*." "Nah," the patient responded. "Not for me." On the next office visit, in walked my patient, carrying two cartons of nonfat frozen yogurt. We spent the next half-hour enjoying my daughter's old discovery and discussing the wonder of new discoveries.

When you are comfortable with the initial changes and do not have more than occasional feelings of deprivation, you are ready to experiment gradually with reducing even more on the saturated-fat biggies. A comfortable goal for the next few weeks might be to cut down further on red meat and processed meat, whole-milk products, egg yolks, fried foods, and saturated oils, to one serving every two weeks. You might, however, have one serving of meat a week, if it is a small portion (2 to 3 ounces), lean and trimmed of fat.

Long-term, work toward cutting your consumption of these high-fat items even further. Many women have found such a change to be a natural evolution, something that takes place without their being conscious of it. If you find yourself feeling deprived, level off. There is no rush, so give yourself adequate time to adjust.

Eating Out

It is not difficult to enjoy delicious *and* healthy meals outside the comfort of your own home. In restaurants, ordering your meal prepared according to your specifications is common practice, and is considered sophisticated. Almost all restaurants offer fish, chicken, and pasta dishes;

grilled, broiled, and steamed vegetables; and low-fat dressings, seasonings, and sauces. Ask the waiter to have the chef limit or eliminate butter and fat in the cooking, and ask that dressings and sauces be served on the side so you can control the amount. Request healthy alternatives—vinegar or lemon instead of a fatty dressing; margarine instead of butter or sour cream.

For those of you who may not know menu terminology, keep in mind that boiled, steamed, broiled, roasted, grilled, and baked foods are usually good, low-fat choices. High-fat preparations, on the other hand, will be given away by such terms as "fried," "creamed," "in cheese sauce," or "casserole." Pâté and quiche are generally fatty. Don't be afraid to ask what the ingredients of a particular dish are or how it is prepared. For dessert, you might order one "for the table"—so everyone can have a taste or two.

As far as airplane meals are concerned, request a low-fat or vegetarian meal when making your flight reservation. Often the food in special meals tastes better than the food in regular meals.

Sugar, Alcohol, Salt, and Caffeine

High sugar intake has never been linked directly to the development of heart disease. But sugar does raise the level of triglycerides and therefore you should cut down on it if you have high triglycerides. Sugar is a simple carbohydrate, and while for heart health it is better to eat sugar than fat, complex carbohydrates—bread, pasta, rice, and potatoes—are far more efficient sources of calories than simple sugar. The major sources of simple sugar, of course, are sweets and desserts—candy, syrups, some beverages, ice cream, pies, cakes, and cookies.

The key word on alcohol consumption is *moderation*. Recent studies have suggested that 1 to 2 ounces of alcohol (the equivalent of 1 to 2 ounces of wine or glasses of beer) increase good cholesterol levels and reduce the risk of heart attack and stroke. Drinking alcohol in greater amounts is not wise, because it tends to increase blood pressure and can have a toxic effect on the heart, liver, and other organs.

Reducing salt (specifically sodium) is important primarily if you have high blood pressure. Simply decreasing salt intake allows many women with hypertension to lower their blood pressure (see chapter 7). There is no evidence that you need to restrict your salt intake if you do not have high blood pressure or heart failure.

Despite several studies suggesting a possible link between caffeine and the risk of heart disease, the connection has never been proven. Caffeine can cause irregular heartbeat in susceptible women, and some authorities believe excess caffeine can make certain individuals more prone to stress. Having recently stopped drinking five or six cups of coffee a day (a habit that began during my internship), I can attest that decreasing one's caffeine intake can be calming. It makes sense to limit your caffeine intake to two or three cups of coffee a day, or the equivalent. Caffeine is found also in colas, chocolate, and nonherbal tea.

HOW TO DECODE FOOD LABELS

Reading and understanding food labels is of course necessary if you are to be conscious of what you eat. Understanding what these labels really mean is not difficult, and it helps you avoid being fooled by misleading terms. There are three parts to a food label:

• Nutrition information per serving. This tells you the serving size, the number of servings per container, the number of calories per serving, and the amount of the three basic food ingredients—protein, carbohydrates, and fat—as well as cholesterol and salt, per serving. Evaluate this information on the basis of *your* anticipated serving size, not solely on what is listed on the label.

• Percentage of the U.S. recommended daily allowances: Amounts are given for protein, vitamins, and minerals.

• Ingredients: These are listed in descending order of weight.

Recently, the Food and Drug Administration has mandated regulations to make food labels easier to read and comprehend. Among the new requirements:

1. Standardized description of a serving, reflecting how much a person is likely to consume. Critics had complained that serving sizes in the past tended to be too small, thus in effect understating the number of calories people probably would consume.

2. Specification of how much of the daily recommended allowance of a nutrient one serving will provide.

3. Listing of values for saturated fat, cholesterol, and total carbohydrates. This information, although often shown in the past, was not required.

4. Translation of grams of fat into calories from fat. Fat had been listed only in grams.

5. Information for recommended daily allowances

based on a 2,500-calorie intake, common among adolescents and active adults, as well as those for a 2,000-calorie diet. In the past, only the latter was taken into account.

6. Gram-to-calorie calculations.

Misleading Labels

Despite the Food and Drug Administration's labeling regulations, many terms used by food manufacturers can be misleading. Be aware of the true meanings of words as they relate to your eating plan, and make your purchases on the basis of nutritional listings, not vague adjectives. Here are a few examples to watch for:

• "Light" and "lite": There are no labeling regulations currently for these words, which are applied freely to many foods. They are used even to describe the appearance or texture of food, not its content.

• "Extra-lean": Products with this on the label must have a fat content of 5 percent or less by weight than a comparable product.

• "Cholesterol-free": This means there are no more than 2 milligrams of cholesterol per serving. Foods with this label can, however, be loaded with saturated or other fat. A cholesterol-free product thus is not always a healthy choice.

• "90% free" or "10% fat": Often found on cold-cut packages, this designation means that 10 percent of the product by weight is fat. But since much of the weight of the meats is from water, they in fact may have more than half of their calories from fat.

• "Nondairy": This indicates only that the product contains no fat from milk. It may be loaded with saturated fats such as coconut oil or palm oil.

Simply by making food label evaluations a routine part of your shopping, you will become more knowledgeable and conscious about food and naturally more aware of the amount of fat you eat.

POTENTIAL PITFALLS

Our notorious inability to maintain a long-term commitment to eating the way we really ought and want to is due to any of a number of factors. Thoughtfulness and attention are the best ways to deal with them successfully.

Automatic eating. The problem with altering eating habits successfully is that most of us eat automatically, not consciously. A conscious eater *thinks* before eating and while eating, whatever gets eaten. Automatic, compulsive eating often is followed by guilt, which leads to more compulsive eating, loss of control, and ultimately resignation to failure.

Paying attention to what and how you eat is vital to success in changing your eating patterns. How you eat is a matter of habit, and as with any change in habit, it takes both time and concentration. So stay aware and be patient with yourself.

Feelings of deprivation. When you feel deprived, you can be derailed easily from thoughtful to compulsive eating. If you really want that steak or slice of pie, make a thoughtful, conscious choice—not a compulsive one—to eat it or not. Above all, be aware not to allow feelings of deprivation to build up. When they do accumulate, they may result in thoughtlessness, compulsive eating, and resignation to failure. Making choices consciously will minimize this possibility.

Cravings. These are the cousins of feelings of deprivation. If you feel a desire strongly enough, indulge it, with thoughtfulness. Such occasional thoughtful indulging never hurt anyone. One of my patients put it perfectly: "When I *do* give in and decide to have that steak, I enjoy the sizzle, the smell, and every damn bite!" Note that a craving can be satisfied with a *small* amount of indulging—a 2- to 3-ounce lean steak, a few spoonfuls of ice cream, and so on—if you put your mind to it.

All-or-none thinking. The idea that you have to be perfect is often the best guarantee of failure. As a patient once told me, "I'm so anxious to be good all the time that I wind up being bad half the time." Seeking perfection, yearning after absolutes, exemplifies compulsive behavior, which needs to be avoided. If you make a mistake, if you veer from your eating plan, live with it, learn from it, be okay about it, and start anew.

Situational problems. Various circumstances may present particular difficulties for keeping alert, aware, and in control. Whatever the specific reasons or surroundings, you can remain in command of yourself and your eating.

Stress. Significant stress, or any emotional upset, may cause you to retreat into automatic, compulsive behavior. It may be difficult to remain thoughtful about food and eating. You must remember to pay attention to yourself in trying times. Stay as aware of your situation as you can, and handle it as best you can.

Social situations. You may feel uncomfortable about ordering special food or not eating the way everyone else is at business or social dinners, parties with friends, or family gatherings. Pressure from friends and family to indulge, and tempting food, do not make things any easier. Again, stay conscious of what you are doing on such occasions. Be creative when you are ordering or selecting food, and tell friends and family that you have decided to be more health-conscious. You might even draw favorable attention to yourself in this way.

Lack of physical activity. This corresponds to a diminished awareness of the body and has adverse effects on eating habits. Regular physical activity gives you an enhanced sense of well-being about your body, how it works and how to maintain it. This is a major impetus to eating properly. Physical activity and good eating habits reinforce each other.

Once you accustom yourself to the changes in how and what you eat, patterns will emerge through which you can stay in alignment with your goals, and modify them if necessary, and remain in control. Remember that you *always* have options—unless you give up. There are rewards if you stick with it until the new way of eating becomes a natural part of your life. Conscious, thoughtful behavior is simply more rewarding and fulfilling than automatic, compulsive behavior.

GETTING STARTED

Write specific, concrete answers to the following:

1. What is my goal for conscious eating in the next week?

2. After choosing from the "Taking Action" section, how will I start?

3. When will I start? If not right now, on what day?

4. How will I stick with my plan? What strategies will I use to keep going?

5. What pitfalls may get in my way?

6. What will I do to handle those pitfalls, or avoid them altogether?

7. When will I assess how I am doing with my goals? What will I do to get back on track if I fall short of my goals (modify goals, join support group, start over)?

RECORDING YOUR PROGRESS

Enter the following information in your notebook:

Date

Did I eat according to plan for breakfast? For lunch? For dinner? For snacks?

Did I stay conscious and thoughtful?

If not, when and how did I go off?

Did any pitfalls come up?

What can I learn from today?

TO SUM UP

1. Eating well is not difficult or complicated if you are willing to follow one rule and keep one commitment: Cut the fat by making simple substitutions, and set aside preconceived notions about food to become a thoughtful eater.

2. A thoughtful eater thinks clearly and objectively about food, and is interested in learning about food and health; allows time for changes in eating habits, is sensibly flexible with eating plans; and experiments to learn what works best.

3. Reaching a total cholesterol level under 200 is a sensible and important goal. Equally important is having your good cholesterol and triglyceride levels checked, and your ratio of total to good (HDL) cholesterol determined. Knowing these values will help you understand whether you have a risk of heart disease and what you can do to decrease that risk.

4. The first step to healthy eating is modifying your diet so that no more than 30 percent of your total calories come from fat. This reduction should help lower cholesterol and control weight. If it does not do the job well enough, try reducing further, for instance to a maximum of 10 or 20 percent fat, or consider a cholesterol-lowering drug.

5. Make suitable substitutions to lower your intake of the fat "biggies": red meat and processed meat, whole-milk products, egg yolks, and saturated oils. There are many alternatives to fit individual tastes. It is best to proceed in stages, and only after you are comfortable with the stage you are in. A reasonable short-term goal would be to cut each of the "biggies" to once a week; a reasonable long-term goal would be to cut each to one serving every other week, or less.

6. Recognize and try to avoid pitfalls that can result in a retreat back to compulsive eating: automatic eating; feelings of deprivation; all-or-none thinking; cravings; and situational problems such as stress, uncomfortable social circumstances, or lack of physical activity.

7. Think before eating, whatever you eat. If you allow

yourself a small treat, do it because you've thought about it, and let it be.

8. Compulsive eating leads to guilt, more compulsive eating, and resignation. Stay aware, make conscious choices, learn from your experiences, and stay with your plan. As Gandhi once said, "We cannot in a moment get rid of the habits of a lifetime."

CHAPTER 6

Heredity and Paragenetics: Genes and Your Mind's View of the Hand You Think You Have Been Dealt

Nothing in life is to be feared. It is only to be understood.
MARIE CURIE

My will shall shape my future. . . . Win or lose, only I hold the key to my destiny.
ELAINE MAXWELL

Clearly, heredity plays an important role in coronary heart disease. Yet heredity should not be confused with irrevocable fate. According to current medical research, the genetic factors related to the development of coronary heart disease are for most people predispositions, not inevitabilities. Atherosclerosis is multifactorial: it is the result of an interaction of multiple predisposing genes and multiple environmental factors (such as smoking). The overall hereditary risk for coronary artery disease is less significant than for several other genetically determined disorders.

A few years ago, several remarkable experiences with patients opened my eyes to a potentially powerful element, sometimes hidden, in the connection between heredity and coronary heart disease. I found that many of my patients had been haunted by their parents' cardiac history, and in particular by the age at which their parents died. Consciously or subconsciously, they had developed a conviction that they would not live beyond that age.

Joan was a sixty-eight-year-old saleswoman who was admitted to the coronary care unit with a heart attack. After reviewing her situation carefully, I told Joan, "Well, there is good news. Your heart attack was minor and the blockage that caused it is in a small artery. Your outlook is very good." Joan stared vacantly at the wall. "Thanks for trying to reassure me, but my time is up and I know it." Stunned, I exclaimed, "Joan, I am not trying to just 'reassure' you! This is really a very minor problem. There is absolutely no medical reason why you shouldn't do just fine!" But my patient was not listening.

To my amazement, Joan did not do well. She developed unpredictable episodes of increase in heart rate. Her blood pressure would suddenly shoot up to alarmingly high levels, for no clear reason. During these episodes she had severe heart rhythm disturbances and required intravenous medication for control. Tests showed no medical reason for these episodes.

One day I was in to see Joan, and I asked how she was feeling. "I'm not going to make it out of here," she told me. "I know it, and you know it too." "I really don't know that at all," I responded. "Why are you so certain?" In a flat, emotionless tone, Joan said, "I'm sixty-eight, and it's my time." "But why would you say that sixty-eight is your time?" I wondered aloud. "You're still young." Joan looked up at me. "My mother died of a heart attack at sixty-eight."

After listening to a careful, detailed explanation of her condition (including angiogram pictures, which showed that the major arteries were clear), and seeing a therapist, Joan finally came to see that sixty-eight wasn't "her time." She was discharged from the hospital and did very well.

This phenomenon of identifying with one's parents is by no means limited to women. One of the most dramatic encounters I have had in medicine was with Alan, a forty-four-year-old policeman. For two years, he had been in an increasing panic about pains that would hop all over his chest as if someone were poking him with a pin. Although these strange symptoms were not due to a heart problem, Alan had been to several cardiologists; all of them had tried, in vain, to reassure him. "I know they are wrong," he said, "and I want a test to prove it." While also reassuring Alan, I told him that if a test would convince him, we would do a stress treadmill. Needless to say, he passed with flying colors. But when I informed him of the results, he maintained that the test was not accurate enough. "I want an angiogram. All the doctors tell me that's the most accurate." I protested that it was unnecessary, but Alan insisted adamantly that he would find "someone, someplace" to administer the test. Very reluctantly, I agreed to do the angiogram.

On the afternoon after the test, I went to Alan's hospital room, where he was asleep. I leaned over him and whispered, "Alan, I have great news! Your arteries are wide open. Not a hint of blockage." He opened his eyes and glared at me, suddenly grabbed my shirt, then pulled me down toward himself and screamed, "You're a liar! You're all liars! I hate all you people. Why the hell won't you tell me the truth!''

Later that day—after both of us had recovered—we had a talk. Alan recalled the time his father discovered that he had failed a high school math test and beat him with a strap. An hour later, Alan's father collapsed; he was rushed to a hospital and pronounced dead of a heart attack—at age forty-four. Once he came to understand the guilt he had about his father's death, Alan's obsession with dying at the same age as his father subsided. His chest pains also disappeared.

Sarah was a patient of mine who became obsessed with her mother's death of a heart attack at age fifty-six. According to Sarah's family, she talked about it incessantly. When she turned fifty-six, she started experiencing chest pains and so had an angiogram. The test showed that her arteries and her heart were normal, but this did not alleviate her fears. A month after the angiogram, Sarah developed a "flu" and after several days became severely short of breath. Despite the fact that she was deteriorating rapidly, Sarah refused her family's pleas to see a doctor and died suddenly. An autopsy showed that she had suffered an overwhelming infection of the heart muscle which had seriously damaged its ability to function (the medical diagnosis was viral myocarditis).

More recently, I was with a group of people listening to a man named Jerry discuss his heart problem. He began very emotionally, by telling us not about himself, but about his father. He was sitting with family and friends near their cabin when suddenly a large snake appeared. Jerry's father ran up an incline to the cabin, ran back down with a rifle, took dead aim at the snake, killed it with one shot, and then fell to the ground. He was dead of a massive heart attack at age sixty-four. For Jerry, who was thirty-seven at the time, heart disease became "my own bugaboo." When he began to tell us *his* story, his tone changed completely. He was almost without emotion as he described a recent year in his life filled with ominously deep psychological depression and anxiety, "like a shadow pursuing me." It culminated in a heart condition—in the year in which he turned sixty-four. Fortunately, Jerry knew a physician whom he respected and whose advice he took. He began a solid program including exercise, stress reduction, and a lowfat diet. Subsequent tests showed that his heart problem regressed dramatically.

These experiences and many others like them have convinced me that in addition to genes themselves, our mind's view of our genes—what I call "paragenetics"—has a major effect on health and longevity. When we believe that our parents' medical history and longevity determines our own health destiny, the belief strongly reinforces any actual genetic factors.

What role do genes play in the development of coronary artery disease? Genetic diseases generally fall into one of three categories: First, chromosomal disorders, which involve the production of excessive or deficient genes; Down's syndrome is such a disorder. Second, simply inherited disorders, which are determined primarily by a single altered, or mutant, gene; sickle-cell anemia, an abnormality affecting red blood cells, is an example. And third, multifactorial disorders, which result from an interaction of multiple genetic and environmental factors; coronary heart disease is an example of this type of disorder. Genetics experts agree that the risk of inheriting a disorder is significantly lower in the last category than in the first two.

The child of a parent with coronary artery disease

inherits one-half of that parent's genes and to that extent is at increased risk. But the chance that a child will inherit the right combination of risk genes decreases as the number of genes necessary to cause that disease increases. Since the precise number of genes responsible for a multifactorial disorder such as coronary heart disease is unknown, the precise genetic risk is very difficult to calculate.

Genetic risk is influenced primarily by two factors. First, the number of immediate family members (parents or siblings) affected. The larger the number of family members with coronary artery disease, the higher the risk. Second, the onset and severity of the disease in family members. The chance that a person will develop coronary heart disease is higher, for instance, if a parent or sibling had a heart problem before age fifty-five.

According to Nobel Prize–winning geneticists Joseph Goldstein and Michael Brown: "In most families that seem genetically predisposed to coronary artery disease by history, *the nature of the genetic factors underlying this predisposition is obscure.* Most patients with coronary artery disease have inherited multiple predisposing genes that *interact with multiple environmental factors* to produce the disease. In these patients *atherosclerosis does not have a single cause*" (italics added). In some patients, Brown and Goldstein go on to say, "coronary artery disease is produced by a single abnormal gene that has a major effect. . . .The most common of these single-gene disorders are those that produce hyperlipidemia [high levels of fat in the blood]." Brown and Goldstein estimate the usual genetic risk for the child of a parent who has had coronary artery disease as 5 to 10 percent. For women, the risk may be even lower.

The most common hereditary factors for coronary heart disease involve the abnormal regulation of lipids, namely fats such as cholesterol, or lipoproteins, the proteins that carry them in the bloodstream to the walls of the arteries. Two doctors, Shea and Nichols, who have studied the role of genes in coronary heart disease, have concluded that a family history for the disease could be explained largely on the basis of known risk factors. In other words, genes cause elevations of cholesterol, blood pressure, and so on, and it is *these* elevated levels that in turn cause atherosclerosis. Research shows that when these risk factors are reduced, health and longevity are affected favorably, regardless of genes.

People at higher risk may have a higher susceptibility to the effects of high cholesterol, high blood pressure, and smoking. Overall:

• A 1-percent reduction in total cholesterol can reduce the risk of coronary heart disease by 2 percent.

• Lowering blood pressure 5 to 6 points (millimeters of mercury) can reduce the risk of a stroke by 40 to 45 percent and the risk of dying from heart disease by 14 percent.

• Even though a smoker has more than twice the heart attack risk of a nonsmoker, quitting dramatically decreases the risk.

Evidence is accumulating that even when genetic factors are to blame for abnormally high blood lipid levels in women, there are other important factors they can control. At a recent American Heart Association meeting, Dr. Joseph Selby discussed the role of genetics and other influences in men and women with the clustering of cardiovascular risk factors known as dyslipemic hypertension (the combination of high lipid levels and hypertension). Dr.

Selby believes "there is evidence for a genetic influence on the clustering of coronary heart disease risk factors, but more important, there is strong evidence that nongenetic influences lead to the expression of the syndrome." Among the principal "nongenetic influences" is significant weight gain in genetically susceptible adults.

TAKING ACTION

If any member of your immediate family has had coronary heart disease, you should evaluate your risk factors carefully. This is particularly important if the disease has struck someone in your family before age fifty-five. Since genetic factors predispose to coronary heart disease largely through risk factors, take stock of the following:

1. Smoking habit
2. Total cholesterol, and LDL (bad) and HDL (good) cholesterol
3. Blood pressure
4. Weight
5. Blood sugar (for diabetes) and triglycerides
6. Life-style (sedentary or active)
7. Stress

Taking action against abnormalities of these risk factors is the key to decreasing your hereditary risk. Specific measures such as going on a low-fat diet, becoming physically active, and handling stress are important. You have a major opportunity to combat coronary heart disease, even if you have a hereditary risk.

The following written exercise may help you obtain

valuable insights into your thoughts and feelings about your heredity and how they may affect your outlook on health and longevity. When you understand self-defeating feelings about what your family health history has meant to you, you will see that these feelings are not based on facts or "the way it has to be." It is important that you actually *do* the exercise, and write out your answers. This should take no more than ten minutes.

1. How long (to what age) do you think you will live?

2. Why do you think you will live to that age? (a) family history or "genes" (b) intuition (c) health habits (d) don't know

3. If they are alive, how old are your father and mother? If they are no longer alive, to what age did they live?

4. Did or do either your father or your mother have a cardiovascular disease?

5. How long (to what age) would you really like to live? Why?

6. Do you think anything can be done to change your health and longevity outlook? (a) yes (b) no (c) don't know
   If so, what?

7. How much impact do you think your thoughts have on your health and longevity? (a) a lot (b) very little (c) don't know
   Why?

8. How much impact do you think changing your thoughts could have on your health and longevity? (a) a lot (b) very little (c) don't know
   Why?

9. Are you willing to reevaluate your thoughts and

feelings about your health and longevity? (a) yes (b) no (c) don't know

Why?

10. Make two columns on a piece of paper. On the left, write five thoughts, feelings, or beliefs about your family medical history and your health and longevity outlook that do not serve you well. On the right, list corresponding alternatives that would serve you better.

How to Interpret Your Answers

1. If you have not answered questions 1 and 5 with a ripe old age like eighty-five or ninety, your expectations are limiting you—unless of course, you are already at a ripe old age.

2. If your answer to question 2 was (a), or possibly (b), and you answered (b) to questions 6 through 9, you demonstrate a sense of resignation about your health and longevity. I suggest that you read or reread chapter 2, on mind-body communication, to understand more fully the role of beliefs in your health.

3. If you answered (a) to questions 6 through 9, you have a positive attitude that will be valuable in accomplishing the goals of good health and longevity. You are ready for the sound, sensible health program described in this book.

4. If the majority of your answers were "don't know," you probably haven't given the subject of heredity and your health outlook much thought. Read or reread chapter 2, to appreciate more fully how the power of the mind affects your health.

POTENTIAL PITFALLS

There are two major potential pitfalls related to heredity and your heart. The first is resignation to what you believe is inevitable, and inaction particularly if there is a history of coronary heart disease in your family. Heredity indicates only a predisposition; a family history of coronary heart disease does not have to be a sentence. A thorough evaluation of your risk factors and correction of abnormalities in them can affect your health outlook favorably.

The second major pitfall is not stopping to consider questions such as those posed above, in the "Taking Action" section. Answering the questions here takes only ten minutes or so. Many people have a resistance to exploring their thoughts and feelings about their health. Such investigation may feel uncomfortable, and it may seem much easier to them to ignore their feelings and beliefs about health and move on. Some people feel especially guilty asking themselves questions about their parents' health and longevity.

The stronger your feelings about not asking yourself questions—and specifically, doing the written exercise above—the more you are likely to benefit from doing it. You will come to realize that you can take more control. This knowledge is vital to your health, so I strongly encourage you to spend those few minutes on the written exercise.

TO SUM UP

1. While heredity does play a role in the development of coronary artery disease, current research indicates that for most people, genetic factors mean a predisposition for—not the inevitability of—atherosclerosis. Coronary heart disease usually results from the interaction of multiple genetic and environmental factors.

2. Genetic risk for coronary heart disease is influenced mainly by the number of immediate family members who have had the disease, by the time of onset and the severity of the disease in them.

3. Your mental outlook on your genetic background can strongly affect actual genetic factors. Your health can be influenced greatly by the mere conviction that your parents' medical history and longevity will inevitably determine your own. And while a negative mental outlook can reinforce negative genetic factors, a positive outlook can counteract them.

4. Research shows clearly that when such risk factors as high cholesterol, high blood pressure, and smoking are corrected, health and longevity are affected favorably—regardless of genetic factors.

5. If any member of your immediate family has had coronary artery disease (especially if before age fifty-five), you should carefully evaluate your potential risk factors. Taking action against these risk factors is the key to decreasing your hereditary risk as well as bolstering your own power and sense of control.

CHAPTER 7

Reducing Three Big Risks: Obesity, High Blood Pressure, and Diabetes

We are indeed much more than we eat, but what we eat can nevertheless help us to be much more than what we are.
ADELLE DAVIS

What really matters is what you do with what you have.
SHIRLEY LORD

Why are such seemingly different topics as obesity, high blood pressure, and diabetes grouped together in one chapter? Because they are very much interrelated and there are similar or identical methods to prevent and/or control them. The combination of the three is widespread—and lethal. It is estimated that 3 million Americans have both high blood pressure (hypertension) and diabetes, and that this combination reduces life expectancy by about one-third. Cardiovascular disease is responsible for 75 percent of these deaths.

The problems of obesity, high blood pressure, and diabetes are particularly important for women, and various investigations have evaluated their effects on women's health. The Framingham Heart Study found that diabetic women weighed more and had higher blood pressure than nondiabetic women. In addition, their triglyceride levels were higher and good cholesterol levels lower than those of nondiabetic women. A Finnish study of newly diagnosed diabetic women determined likewise that they were more obese and had higher triglyceride and lower good cholesterol levels than nondiabetic women. While the diabetic women did not have high blood pressure, 60 percent of them were taking medication for it.

OBESITY

Obesity is the common denominator. The Framingham Heart Study found that as weight rises and falls, so too do blood pressure and blood sugar (the principal measure for diabetes). Obesity leads to increased resistance in the arteries, which in turn leads to high blood pressure and increased resistance to insulin, which in turn leads to diabetes, high triglycerides, and low good cholesterol. Dr. William Castelli, director of the study, has described this characteristic pattern of obesity, which some have called "syndrome X": "When you put the 'spare tire' on at the waist, you produce a different kind of LDL, much more atherogenic [causing atherosclerosis]. You raise your blood pressure and increase your lipids." In the Framingham study, high blood pressure was three times as prevalent among heavier women than among those weighing less, and Dr. Castelli estimates that overweight women develop diabetes at twice the rate of others. Additional recent research has attributed as much as 70 percent of coronary heart disease among women to their being overweight.

Fran was a thirty-two-year-old obese woman who was referred to me for evaluation after she had experienced pain on the right side of her chest and severe palpitations for several months. Fortunately, she did not have a coronary artery problem; her diagnosis was mitral valve prolapse, a common and generally benign condition whose troubling symptoms may include chest pains, palpitations, and shortness of breath (see chapter 9). I explained to Fran that she was in no immediate danger of a heart attack and that I could prescribe some medication to make her feel better.

However, her blood pressure was high, her triglycerides very elevated, and her good cholesterol too low. I told Fran that while she was not in any immediate danger, she might have more significant heart problems when she was older. The false alarm proved to be a big motivation. Fran joined a weight reduction program, lost forty pounds and kept them off. As a result, both her blood pressure and her lipid levels improved.

Fran's success story is more often the exception than the rule. Studies show that obesity is more of a risk factor for heart disease in women than in men, and is disproportionately high among women. A recent survey found that 33 to 40 percent of the adult women were trying to lose weight, compared with 20 to 24 percent of the men; another 28 percent of the women were seeking to maintain their weight. Many of the women surveyed, it should be added, wanted to lose weight for the wrong reasons, while many obese women had given up on trying to lose weight.

A panel of experts on obesity recently reported that "for most people, achieving body weights and shapes presented in the media is not a reasonable or appropriate goal." The panel urged people not to set a specific short-term weight-loss target, but instead to adopt a longer view that emphasizes a healthy life-style, including exercise and sound nutrition. One panelist, endocrinologist C. Wayne Callaway, commented that "we are in an epidemic of inappropriate dieting." The panel agreed with studies indicating that obesity is disproportionately high among women.

All too often, a woman's attempts at weight control are a repeated series of failures. Helen provides a typical example. When I first saw her, she was a 240-pound hypertensive diabetic who had spent a lifetime on rice diets, water diets, grapefruit diets, liquid diets, starvation diets, repeatedly losing and regaining "thousands of pounds." Finally she gave up. "It's hopeless," she told me, staring vacantly at the floor. "I'm just not capable of keeping the weight off. I've spent a fortune on it. I'm totally frustrated and I don't want to think about it anymore. If you tell me I have to start another diet, I won't be able to keep seeing you." I asked her, "How would you like to go on a health program—not a diet but a program—that will make you feel healthier than you have ever felt before?" Helen looked at me skeptically and said, "I'm willing to listen, but I want to warn you, I've already heard all the hype." The program I outlined for her, and for all of my overweight patients, is the one presented below.

TAKING ACTION

The best approach to achieving and maintaining a healthy weight has four basic components. None of them involves "being on a diet."

Understanding and modifying your relationship to food. This will enable you to be in control rather than under the control of compulsions or rigid and unrealistic goals. Eating without thinking, urgently weighing yourself every day, setting perfectionist goals are followed inevitably by depression and hopelessness if and when you slip and binge. A sensible relationship to food will release you from the typical up-and-down dieting cycle once and for all.

The importance of freeing yourself from yo-yo dieting goes beyond self-esteem. A recent study published in *The New England Journal of Medicine* concluded that such dieting increases the risk of heart disease by as much as 30 percent. Among subjects in the study, those who lost 10 percent or more of their body weight three or more times and then regained it had their risk of coronary artery disease increase by 50 percent.

Changing your attitude to food is not yet another diet plan. People who emphasize dieting are treating only the symptoms, according to author Dr. Janet Greeson, who has managed not to regain the 150 pounds she lost more than eighteen years ago. "Diets are not really treating the person, and so if you focus on food as the problem . . . you are not successful . . . because food is not the problem. The problem is the feelings a person associates with food." Understanding how your mind affects your eating habits is crucial.

"If you eat when you are not hungry," as Dr. Greeson says, "you know that something else is going on." You have to ask why you are eating or overeating. To comprehend why and under what circumstances you overeat, keep a detailed diary of what, when, and how you eat every day for the next five days. Consider especially the following:

• What is your eating pattern? Do you continually nibble? Do you binge at particular hours or on particular occasions (at times of stress or emotional strain)? Do situations that evoke such negative feelings as loneliness, self-doubt, low self-esteem, powerlessness, anger, or loss of control cause you to binge? Do you do reasonably well during the day, but at night absentmindedly (significant word) turn to food while watching television?

• Overeating is a common way to attempt to avoid unwanted, at times scary, emotions; in this sense it becomes a "solution." Writing careful notes about the times and circumstances that seem to generate an impulse to binge will help you anticipate them in the future, understand them, and develop a successful strategy to deal with them.

• If you overate or binged, how did you feel afterward? Did you feel guilty, frightened, depressed, hopeless? Do your emotions contribute to the problem by convincing you that you are flawed and doomed to failure? Does overeating make you feel there is something fundamentally "not okay" about you? Remember, it is no big deal to slip; a binge by itself never hurt anyone. The real danger of a binge is the guilt attached, which leads to loss of control (including more compulsive eating) and ultimately feelings of failure and resignation.

• What is it that overeating is preventing you from experiencing about yourself or in your life? Identifying such matters will bring them into the light, where they can be dealt with in a healthy way. Writing about otherwise hidden feelings and communicating them (through, for example, a support group; see below) are invaluable paths to self-discovery. You will be surprised and relieved to find that your dark secrets aren't nearly as terrible or frightening as you might have feared. While communicating may not always be an easy process, it is without a doubt worthwhile.

Enjoying what you eat by becoming a conscious eater. This will help you select healthy and satisfying food—including some of your favorites—rather than limit you to rigid calorie-cutting and self-deprivation.

Chapter 5 emphasized the importance of being a thoughtful eater: considering clearly and objectively what and how you eat, being knowledgeable about what you eat, and allowing for slips and binges. Being knowledgeable about what you eat means being able to select healthy, *satisfying* food. By learning about food, you can make simple substitutions in your diet that will keep you feeling satisfied while helping you achieve a desirable weight. The key here has been mentioned before: Cut the fat. Cutting fat decreases not only total cholesterol but calories as well; an ounce of fat has more than twice the calories of an ounce of protein or carbohydrate. For the best ways to lower the fat in your diet, see chapter 5.

Being a conscious eater does not mean you have to give up tasty food. You can include some of your old favorites, in modest amounts, in your overall eating plan. Deprivation, keep in mind, simply does not work long-term; it results in compulsive overeating for most dieters. If you really want a particular food, have it—in a small amount once every week or two. Learn to eat in moderation by having smaller servings. This may be difficult at first, but you will find that it cuts down on calories and gives you a sense of control.

There are other ways to apply conscious eating:

• Eat fresh ingredients, prepared simply. You will find that the best meals for you involve the least preparation, and you can follow this principle whether eating at home or eating out.

• Seek out a market that carries interesting varieties of produce, fresh fish, pasta, and condiments.

• Experiment with eating patterns to find one that works best for you, and stick with it. Be conscious of the scheduling and makeup of meals and snacks, and the times and circumstances in which you are prone to bingeing.

Keep in mind that the longer you eat healthy, satisfying food, the better you will feel and the less often you will crave rich or fatty food.

Exercising regularly. While jogging in a park not long ago, I ran into a former patient, a self-proclaimed "fatty." She looked great as she walked briskly in a bright jogging suit, and I couldn't resist asking her about her appearance. "I've lost thirty pounds and kept it off for a year now," she told me. "And I really feel terrific." "How did you do it?" I asked. "Are you on some new diet?" Just the opposite, she said: "I simply went off diets and started walking every other day. Those diets were so unsatisfying. I couldn't stand living that way. Every time a diet ended, I pigged out and blew up like a balloon. Now all I do is walk, and stay away from fat. Fat is the enemy, not food."

Physical activity is a powerful weapon in weight control for several reasons: It burns calories, it contributes to positive feelings and thus reduces the stresses and emotions that cause overeating, and it restores a consciousness of the body, which overweight people tend to lose. Simple exercise allows you to reclaim yourself physically and thereby strengthens your motivation to achieve and maintain a healthy weight.

The results of a study conducted recently at Baylor University are telling. The 150 subjects were all in weight-loss programs, 50 dieting, 50 exercising, and 50 dieting and exercising. Those who only dieted lost the most weight initially, but they regained all the weight in two years. Those who dieted and exercised lost less weight than those who only dieted, but they regained most of the weight in two years. Those who only exercised lost the least weight initially, *but* they kept it off *and continued to lose weight*. The initial results, then, had a limited benefit. Dieting and exercise have different functions and effects. Exercise, for one, builds muscle, which weighs more than fat; the people who only dieted lost more weight at first simply because they did not engage in muscle-building exercise.

"Exercise leads to a sense of well-being, which helps people feel in control of their lives and helps them control their weight," says psychologist John Foreyt, director of the Nutrition Research Clinic at Baylor. He goes on to say that while dieting "gives people an emotional high from temporary weight loss, the more you emphasize diet only, the more likely you are to yo-yo, and the harder it is in the long run to keep the weight off."

Getting support for yourself. This can come from family, friends, and/or a support group.

Enlisting your family means asking them to help shop for food, prepare and serve meals, and clean up afterward, as a patient of mine discovered. Kate, forty-eight years old, was overweight and had been suffering from chest pains. Tests, however, reassured her that there was no evidence of a heart problem. I talked with Kate, an office manager, about how she did a beautiful job of organizing her staff at work, but seemed to feel she had to do everything herself at home. When Kate decided to take better care of herself and lose weight, she called a meeting of her husband and three teenage children. She told them she wanted their support in her resolve to become healthier and presented a rotation system for food shopping, cooking, serving, and cleaning up after meals. They agreed that the plan was fair and reasonable—and Kate lost twenty-five pounds.

These hints may prove helpful around the house, and around food:

- Keep out of harm's way: stay out of the kitchen unless you are preparing meals.
- Try not to eat while you are cooking.
- Set specific times for snacks, and choose healthy, low-calorie foods—a bowl of veggies or some fruit instead of potato chips or cookies, for instance.
- Drink a glass of water every two hours or so; this is a healthy way to decrease your appetite.
- Write down a list of healthy, low-fat, low-calorie foods before going to the supermarket, to help keep you on track. Do not shop for food when you are hungry.

STRUCTURED WEIGHT-LOSS PROGRAMS

Joining a structured weight-loss program can be invaluable—especially for women. Such a program provides you with a supportive environment and people who both understand and share your struggle with overeating. In this setting, you can hear other people talk about themselves and their feelings and emotions about eating, which may be relevant to your own. A solidly structured program will support you to become stronger in your resolve and enhance your understanding about your relationship to food. You can be more honest with yourself, and when you feel you may be slipping, you can ask for help. And you can learn important new techniques and strategies about food and conscious eating.

WHAT IS OBESITY?

While the term *obesity* implies an excess of fat tissue, the meaning of *excess* is somewhat hard to define. Aesthetic considerations aside, obesity can be defined as any degree of excess fat tissue that imparts a health risk. The cutoff between "normal" and "obese" is something of an approximation. According to the Framingham Heart Study, a weight 20 percent above the desirable level constitutes a health risk, or obesity. A National Institutes of Health panel on obesity agreed with this definition. Using this criterion, some 30 to 40 percent of American adult women, and 20 to 30 percent of American adult men, are obese.

From a health standpoint, certain patterns of obesity may be less desirable than others. Fat deposits around the waist and sides, for instance, as evidenced by a high ratio of waist to hip measurement, are associated with a greater health risk than fat deposits at the hips.

Healthy, desirable, or ideal weights are based on averages for people with normal life expectancies, and vary of course according to height. Measurement of relative weight—involving an average range for height and age—is useful particularly to allow for differences in build. The proportion of weight, and of obesity, is often expressed by the body mass index, or BMI, which is body weight divided by height.

Relative weight and BMI indicate the degree of excess fat; excess pounds, however, may be either muscle or fat tissue. Nevertheless, these measurements have matched up well with the risk predictions for the adverse effects of obesity on health and longevity. More precise assessments of obesity can be made with measurements of body density.

POTENTIAL PITFALLS

Losing weight, as well as maintaining a healthy weight, is undeniably difficult for many people. Some women face particular pitfalls, which if not recognized and dealt with consciously, can go a long way:

Using food as an outlet for anger, frustration, or feelings of being ignored. Eating can seem to calm emotions that appear to lack other outlets. In particular, heavy, fatty, or rich foods can make you numb and dull your painful or negative feelings. When you want to overeat but don't, emotions surface that you may not want to feel. Remember that these are the very emotions that will provide clues to gaining control and freeing yourself. If you are anxious, calm yourself; it *is* safe for these emotions to arise, if you accept them. They are never as terrible as you think they will be.

Using food to celebrate. For some women, parties and other gatherings, vacations, and similar happy occasions are a time for "letting go"—and overeating. Anticipate these events and decide *in advance* how you will eat sensibly and have fun without overindulging.

Using food as a quick fix for boredom, depression, or fatigue. Foods high in sugar give the illusion of providing solace when you are bored or blue, and energy when you are exhausted. While eating such foods may make you feel better for an hour or two, you will then face a quick drop in blood sugar and a craving for more sugar. Satisfying that craving means excess weight gain, which in the long turn will add to depression and fatigue. Ask yourself and your support system what else you can do in your life to feel less bored, depressed, or fatigued. The answers could prove interesting and even exciting.

Unconscious nibbling. The simplest antidote for this, of course, is to avoid being around food except when you are shopping for it or preparing or eating meals. It also helps not to keep unhealthy foods in the house.

Food often distracts us from problems and unwanted feelings. But avoiding feelings only perpetuates them. Understanding what you are feeling when you overeat may be an enormous relief, and it may lead to solutions that seem impossible otherwise. To find practical and effective ways of understanding and dealing with your emotions, read chapter 4.

HIGH BLOOD PRESSURE

Hypertension, or high blood pressure, is largely a hereditary condition, but it is related to obesity in many women. Most authorities define hypertension as a blood pressure reading that is consistently (in three consecutive readings) above 140/90. The first value here (140), the systolic, represents pressure on the arteries during heart contractions, while the second (90), the diastolic, represents pressure between contractions. If the systolic value is elevated, there is excess tension on the arteries during each heart contraction; if the diastolic value is elevated, there is excess tension on them between heart contractions. An elevation of either is a risk: increased tension on the arteries can lead to stroke, heart attack, and kidney disease.

In addition to controlling your weight, what can you do to minimize the risk of high blood pressure? First, cut down on your salt intake. Many people eat much more salt (specifically, sodium) than necessary, and although the extent to which decreased salt intake will lower blood pressure varies among individuals, a good goal to aim for is 1 to 2 grams a day rather than a typical 6 to 12. The easiest ways to reduce the amount of salt in your diet are to not add it while cooking or at the table; to substitute fresh foods for processed foods, such as canned soups, which usually are loaded with salt; and to avoid such high-salt items as processed meats, frozen dinners, chips, and fast foods. While this may not protect you from high blood pressure completely, it can help.

BODY FAT TESTS AND BATHROOM SCALES

Periodically weighing yourself on a bathroom scale generally is adequate for assessing your amount of excess fat. Just remember that the scale can be deceptive. For instance, say you have been eating a low-calorie diet for two weeks without exercising and the scale shows you lost x pounds. Most of what you lost is not fat, but water, plus some muscle mass. You may be carrying nearly as much body fat as before. If you had been on the same diet and had been exercising as well, the scale would indicate that you had lost less weight; you would be building muscle (which weighs more than fat) as you lost body fat. This, indeed, is the desired result, yet the scale reading may be discouraging.

Some diet centers and health clubs use tests of body fat to give you a better, perhaps more encouraging, idea of what's going on in your body. You may want to be tested, out of curiosity or out of a desire to be urged into doing more exercise, if you have excess body fat. This is not necessary, I think, if you stay clear and objective about what is happening when you weigh yourself on the bathroom scale.

Do not become a scale fanatic, weighing yourself several times a day, praising or scolding yourself with each little change. Once a week is sufficient, so you don't get caught up in the minor fluctuations that occur normally. When you weigh yourself, do so always at the same time of day. Your weight may fluctuate by several pounds over the course of twenty-four hours.

Keep in mind that bathroom scales differ, as does their accuracy. Whether you have a dial scale, typically inexpensive and sturdy, or an easy-to-read digital model, it may be less accurate than the scale in your doctor's office. The major purpose of home scales is to show you *changes* in your weight, and thus their consistency is more important than their accuracy. If you are thinking of buying a scale, test its consistency by weighing yourself several times in close succession. Shift your weight from side to side—that should not affect the reading. Make sure you can read the numbers easily. If possible, compare your weight on the scale with the reading on a trusted one, for instance the one at your doctor's office.

The effects of stress on blood pressure also vary with the individual. Dr. Robert Eliot has found that there are two ways in which people react to stress: hot and cold responses. Dr. Herbert Benson's research has also found that relaxation techniques lower blood pressure (see chapter 4 for details). Last, but not least, exercise also decreases stress and may have additional benefits in controlling blood pressure.

It is clear that heightened emotions raise blood pressure temporarily, and there is evidence that stress may contribute to persistent high blood pressure. According to Dr. Leonard Syme of the University of California at Berkeley, people with hypertension "seem to be faced with demanding social situations in which aspirations are blocked, in which meaningful human intercourse is restricted, and in which the outcome of important events is often uncertain." Other researchers have noted that high blood pressure is more common in societies where change is the norm, where people are mobile and insecure in their jobs, and where anxiety never seems to be resolved.

Job stress has been a specific target for study. People who hold high-stress jobs have demonstrated higher average blood pressures than people employed otherwise. A recent study of 200 people in various occupations in New York City revealed that those in high-stress jobs not only had higher blood pressure, but also more frequently suffered from a thickening of the heart wall (the typical response of the heart to hypertension). High-stress jobs are those which demand careful attention to detail but give little latitude for decision making and little personal satisfaction. These jobs seem to take the greatest toll on workers' health.

Another recent study, on preventing hypertension, assessed various methods—weight reduction, limitation of salt intake, stress management, nutritional supplementation—for lowering blood pressure in 2,182 men and women. By losing only ten pounds, several people in the study brought their elevated blood pressure down to the normal range. Subjects in the weight reduction group exercised, most of them by walking for forty-five minutes four or five times a week. Those who cut down their salt intake also lowered their blood pressure. According to researcher Dr. Jeffrey Cutler, "you can get this effect by [having patients] reduce their salt intake from one and a half teaspoons . . . to one teaspoon a day." Stress management and nutritional supplementation did not reduce blood pressure significantly in this study.

DIABETES

Twice as many women as men over age forty-five suffer from diabetes, and women with diabetes who have a heart attack are at a higher risk of dying than diabetic men or nondiabetic women who have a heart attack. Diabetes is a disorder in which the body is unable to use sugar (in medical terminology, glucose) properly. This is because of insufficient production of the hormone insulin (needed to transport sugar from the bloodstream into body tissues) by specialized beta cells in the pancreas, or because of resistance by the tissues to insulin. Type 1, or juvenile, diabetes, due to the insufficient production of insulin, starts in youth and requires insulin treatment for control; more common is type 2 non-insulin-dependent, or adult-onset diabetes, caused by tissue resistance to insulin. Eighty to ninety percent of adult-onset diabetics are obese. It is believed that obesity induces a resistance to insulin, which eventually leads to exhaustion of insulin-producing cells in the pancreas. There is a genetic susceptibility for adult-onset diabetes. However, many authorities believe that an environmental factor usually initiates the disease. Forty percent of siblings and one-third of the offspring of diabetics eventually develop some form of diabetes.

Diabetes is diagnosed upon evaluation of an individual's blood sugar metabolism. This is done by measuring the blood sugar after a two-hour fast or establishing a so-called glucose (sugar) tolerance curve. A blood sugar level of 140 or more after a two-hour fast, or an abnormal glucose tolerance curve indicates diabetes. By age fifty, about one woman in five has abnormal glucose metabolism. This increases to almost one in three by age seventy.

The risk of diabetes may be reduced by two simple dietary methods, namely, decreasing intake of refined *simple* carbohydrates (sugars) and increasing intake of *complex* carbohydrates (in the form of pasta, rice, bread). Eating simple sugars causes a sudden surge of glucose in the bloodstream; this triggers the release of large amounts of insulin and stresses a system that is already defective. Eating a diet high in complex carbohydrates, by contrast, reduces insulin levels.

A recent study from Harvard University showed that exercise may avert diabetes. Of 22,000 subjects—all male physicians—the risk of diabetes over a five-year period was 42 percent lower among those who exercised five times a week than among those who exercised less than once a week. But exercising even only once a week reduced the risk by 23 percent. "Our results suggest that diabetes can now be added to the list of conditions that can be prevented by physical activity," says Dr. Jo Ann Manson, one of the

Harvard researchers. These findings were independent of weight fluctuations. In fact, overweight men who exercised once a week had a risk for diabetes 40 percent lower than that for men who exercised less frequently. According to Dr. Manson, exercise may lessen the risk of diabetes by decreasing fat tissue and increasing tissue sensitivity to insulin. Of course, if weight control, dietary changes, and exercise are not sufficient to avert or control diabetes, medication is necessary.

GETTING STARTED

Write specific, concrete answers to the following:

1. What is my goal for the next week? Will I start a diary of my eating habits, develop a concrete eating plan, join a support group, enlist my family, begin exercising, or do something else?

2. What are my goals for each of the next three weeks after that?

3. When will I start? If not right now, on what day?

4. How will I stick with my plan? What strategies will I use to keep going?

5. What pitfalls may get in my way?

6. What will I do to handle these pitfalls, or avoid them altogether?

7. When will I assess how I am doing with my goals? What will I do to get back on track if I fall short of my goals (modify goals, join support group, start over)?

RECORDING YOUR PROGRESS

Enter the following information in a notebook:

Date
Did I stay with my plan today?
If not, when and how did I go off?
Did any pitfalls come up?
What can I learn from today?

TO SUM UP

1. Obesity, high blood pressure, and diabetes are very closely interrelated. The combination is widespread and lethal, reducing life expectancy by one-third. These disorders are particularly important for women.

2. Weight is often the decisive factor: as it rises or falls, so too do blood pressure and blood sugar. Obesity commonly is accompanied by hypertension, diabetes, high triglycerides, and low good (HDL) cholesterol levels.

3. Achieving and maintaining a healthy weight need not involve "being on a diet." Instead, it depends on: understanding and modifying your relationship to food; enjoying what you eat by substituting healthy, satisfying food (including some of your favorites) rather than rigidly cutting calories and depriving yourself; exercising regularly; and getting assistance for yourself by joining a good support group.

4. High blood pressure can be minimized with weight control, and by limiting salt intake. Lowering stress also can be helpful.

5. Diabetes can be offset by weight control, by limiting simple sugar intake and increasing complex carbohydrate intake. Exercising regularly is useful as well.

6. Major potential pitfalls to achieving and maintaining a healthy weight are using food as an outlet for emotions, as a quick fix, or to celebrate; and unconsciously nibbling.

CHAPTER 8

Smoking: Why You Can't Quit, and How You Can

Supposing you have tried and failed again and again. You may have a fresh start any moment you choose.
MARY PICKFORD

You need to claim the events of your life to make yourself yours.
FLORIDA SCOTT MAXWELL

When I was a boy growing up in New York City, our next-door neighbor was Mrs. Levy, a heavy cigarette smoker. One day I heard the loud siren of an ambulance on the street below our building. Men dressed in white entered Mrs. Levy's apartment and after a few minutes carried her out on a stretcher. I asked my mother what was happening, and she told me that Mrs. Levy had had a heart attack and was being taken to the hospital. Mrs. Levy returned home after a couple of weeks, and my family went to visit her. When we walked into her bedroom, we found it filled with smoke. An ashtray was full of cigarette butts, and she was deeply inhaling a lit cigarette. My mother said, "Wasn't your heart attack scary enough to convince you to stop?" Mrs. Levy looked up at my mother and said, "I would rather die than stop smoking!" One week later, she was found dead in her apartment.

Despite that frightening childhood experience, I started to smoke while I was a teenager. By the time I went to college, I had become a pack-a-day smoker—choosing the same brand of cigarettes as my parents smoked. The stresses of my schooling increased, and so did my smoking. I was up to one and a half packs a day by my second year of medical school.

My experience was typical. Most smokers begin early in life. Statistics show that 80 percent of smokers who were born since 1935 started smoking before age twenty-one, and more than 50 percent before age eighteen. Hearing of and understanding the dangers of cigarette smoking seems not to be an effective deterrent for teenagers. Surveys have shown that 90 percent of teenagers who smoke know that it is harmful to their health.

The warnings about the hazards of smoking *have* had an effect on adult smokers. Currently about 40 million Americans are former smokers. Yet most of these former smokers are men, and it is only the number of men who smoke that has decreased substantially in recent years. In 1965, about half of American men smoked; today, according to the Centers for Disease Control, it is down to a quarter. The picture is very different for women: Not only are fewer women than men quitting, but the number of teenage girls who smoke is increasing.

There are several reasons for this. For one, teenage girls are a major target for advertising by the tobacco industry. For another, teenagers are susceptible if they are from families in which one or both parents smoke, and teenage girls especially so. According to the Mayo Clinic: "Because more mothers now smoke than in past generations, more of their daughters mimic their smoking behavior."

Smoking is the single most serious health concern for women. It is, to quote the U.S. surgeon general, "the most important of the known modifiable risk factors for coronary heart disease in the United States," and this even may be more true for women than for men. The Framingham Heart Study has warned that a fifty-five-year-old woman who smokes is in more danger of having a heart attack than a fifty-five-year-old male smoker.

Despite these depressing statistics, however, there are grounds for optimism—if you stop smoking. Several studies have found that when a person quits smoking, the risk of heart disease and lung disease decreases substantially. Research at the Mayo Clinic indicates that the risk of a heart attack decreases within a year after a person stops smoking. Other research has shown that ten years after quitting, the risk for heart disease is about the same as if a person had never smoked. A recent study from Australia is even more encouraging. It found that only three years after quitting, ex-smokers had the same risk of a heart attack as people who never had smoked. In reporting this study, Dr. Timothy Ingall concluded that "the clear message is this: Stop smoking. There is benefit to stopping, whether one is thirty or eighty."

Even after a heart attack there is benefit to stopping. Angiogram X-ray studies that visualize the coronary arteries demonstrate that quitting smoking exerts a protective effect against the formation of new atherosclerotic plaque, even in patients with clear-cut coronary disease. On the other hand, according to German investigator Dr. Peter Nikutta, "Cigarette smoking . . . significantly accelerated the formation of new coronary lesions." Studies show that after a heart attack, quitting smoking helps reduce the risk of a fatal new attack or sudden death by 20 to 50 percent.

Clearly, then, there are good reasons for women to stop smoking. First and foremost is that for women, smoking is the most important risk factor for a heart attack, and quitting decreases that risk significantly. Second, by not smoking, women can set an example for teenagers and younger women (and men) who are current or would-be smokers. Third, quitting means eliminating the environmental dangers smoking presents for other people.

EFFECTS OF SMOKING ON CIRCULATION

Cigarette smoke has several immediately harmful effects on the heart and blood vessels. It releases substances that increase blood pressure and heart rate and constrict blood vessels. Tobacco smoke contains carbon monoxide, which when inhaled binds to hemoglobin, taking the place of oxygen, and thereby decreases the availability of oxygen to the heart.

Smoking promotes the long-term development of atherosclerosis. It increases the clumping and stickiness of blood platelet elements, and thus contributes to the deposit of cholesterol in the arteries. Cigarette smokers have lower good cholesterol levels, and the consequent lipid imbalance promotes cholesterol deposits in the blood vessel walls. As a result, smoking is associated with strokes as well as heart attacks. According to the American Heart Association, smokers may be at two or three times greater risk of having a stroke than nonsmokers. In addition, smokers have a greater risk of peripheral vascular disease than do nonsmokers. They may experience leg or thigh pain with exercise, and even suffer gangrene of the foot.

Smoking can also result in premature heart attacks. Cigarette smoke injures the inner lining of the arteries, and that injury, together with increased platelet adhesiveness, increased levels of fibrinogens (which are involved in clotting), and decreased clotting time, all strengthen the likelihood of thrombosis, or blood clot. Tobacco smoke also can bring about spasm of the arteries. All these effects increase the possibility of a heart attack.

Evidence now shows unequivocally that cigarette smoke is hazardous to nonsmokers exposed to it. The American Heart Association has found "overwhelming" proof that so-called passive smoking causes tens of thousands of deaths from heart disease each year in the United States. More specifically, it is estimated that spending an hour in a smoke-filled room is equivalent to smoking one cigarette, and that after two hours, the level of carbon monoxide in the blood of exposed nonsmokers doubles. When one spouse in a household smokes, the nonsmoking spouse has risk of heart disease almost one-third higher than either spouse in a nonsmoking household. This is all the more important because about half of all children in the United States live in homes with at least one smoker. As part of a concerted effort to curb this "major preventable cause of cardiovascular disease and death," the American Heart Association recently issued a strong position paper. "Environmental tobacco smoke [should] be treated as an environmental toxin," it concluded, "and ways to protect

the public from this health hazard should be developed."
The AHA report strongly supported the establishment of
smoke-free environments in the home, and in public build-
ings and the workplace. It more recently has been supple-
mented by a report from the Environmental Protection
Agency which concluded that passive smoking kills up to
53,000 people per year nationwide—including 37,000 who
die of heart disease.

Where does all this information leave you, if you are
among the estimated 70 to 90 percent of smokers who want
to quit smoking but just can't? Of course quitting is difficult; smoking is a multifaceted problem with physiological,
psychological, and sociological components. If you smoke,
you maintain a certain level of nicotine in your blood. If
you have not had a cigarette for several hours, the level
decreases and you may become irritable and nervous. You
"need a cigarette," and smoking serves to calm you and
relieve your stress. You may find that cigarettes produce
the surge of energy necessary to wake you or keep you
functioning at a high level of intensity. Nicotine is a stimu-
lant with an effect like that of adrenaline; your heart rate
and blood pressure increase while you are smoking. You
may use cigarettes as a prop, something to put in your
hands when you are nervous. They provide a form of dis-
traction and may give you a feeling of security.

Smokers light up when they are stressed, tired, angry,
bored. In fact, cigarettes seem to go well with everything—
eating, drinking, working, driving, watching TV. Smoking
becomes not just a diversion, but a way of dealing with and
relating to life. For many smokers, the long-standing use of
cigarettes in ordinary situations convinces them they cannot cope without smoking.

Whatever the difficulties they faced, millions of Americans have kicked the smoking habit—and so can you. It doesn't matter whether or not you previously have tried to quit but failed. Most people who ultimately quit were unsuccessful in their initial attempts. Your success depends on two factors: how motivated you are to quit, and how well prepared. Motivation develops when you are sick and tired enough once and for all to do something about it.

One of my patients, a fifty-three-year-old homemaker, had been a two-pack-a-day smoker since she was sixteen. Marge had serious heart disease and was becoming increasingly short of breath. We had talked for months about her quitting. I had warned her about the specific types of damage that cigarettes were doing to her body. I had told her about the environmental dangers of cigarette smoke to her two teenage children, and about the studies showing that children of smokers were more than twice as likely to take up smoking than children in nonsmoking households, because of the messages they were getting from their parents that it was okay to smoke. All in vain.

One day Marge came to the office and announced that she had had enough. "You know what," she said, "I don't even enjoy smoking anymore. It's just a lousy habit. I'm sick of making myself sick and risking my kids' health. I'm quitting now! What's the best way to do it?"

Making the commitment to quit is critical; planning and following through on your commitment are equally important. Not everyone can quit cold turkey. Although the majority of former smokers say they quit without help, most of these are men who prefer to go it alone and tough it out. The remainder of this chapter will provide you with some useful and proven ways to stick with your plan.

Not only will quitting be the single most important thing you can do for your own health, but it also may be invaluable to the health of others in your life. Remember, as mentioned before, that most people succeed in making a clean break only after several attempts. Previous failures to quit are viewed best as partial success; they indicate that you are on the right track. "If it doesn't work the first time, or the second or the third," says Clifford Carr, a smoking cessation researcher at UCLA, "it does work on the fourth or fifth try. [People] get better at it." You *can* overcome your obstacles to quitting.

TAKING ACTION

There is no ideal way to quit smoking, and what works for one person may not work for another. The following strategies are intended as tools to help you develop the plan that works best for you.

Assess your motivation. The single most important ingredient in a stop-smoking strategy is your commitment, even though you know quitting may not be easy. To assess the strength of your commitment, answer these questions honestly: Are you *really* ready to quit now? (A maybe counts as a no here.) If you aren't ready, why not? What tools and/or support will you need to maximize your success? Will you go cold turkey, or minimize the withdrawal symptoms? Considering these questions will help you to pick and choose from the suggestions offered below.

Understand withdrawal. You may experience physical withdrawal symptoms for three to ten days (even more, for some smokers). These may occur "predictably," at particular hours or at certain events (on awakening, after meals, during coffee breaks, while working or driving) or randomly throughout the day. When withdrawal symptoms manifest themselves, remember that they will pass; as days go by, you will feel better. Marking days off the calendar can help during the initial period; as will reminding yourself that you are committed to no longer needing cigarettes and that the intensity of these urges will decrease soon.

Inform others. Tell your family and friends of your intention to stop smoking, and the day you intend to begin. Explain why you have chosen to quit, and ask for their support and encouragement.

Set a date to quit, and prepare for it. It is usually best to decide on a particular date within the next two or three weeks. While awaiting the magic day:

• Write a list of all the reasons you are choosing to quit. Review this list on the day you quit smoking and periodically during the first few weeks.

• Keep a diary for several days, recording when and under what circumstances you smoked, how smoking felt, and what, if anything, you got out of the cigarette. Michael Ericksen, a former smoker who runs stop-smoking classes at the M. D. Anderson Cancer Center, says that considering such causes and effects tells smokers "exactly where smoking fits into their lives." You may be surprised by what you find about your smoking habits. According to the American Cancer Society, most smokers really crave only five or six of the cigarettes they smoke. Smokers who can cut down to ten a day may be ready to quit altogether, says Ericksen.

• Change routines. Switch to a brand whose taste or packaging is less appealing than your brand's, and whose amount of nicotine is lower. Buy cigarettes by the pack instead of by the carton. Smoke only half of each cigarette, and gradually reduce the number of cigarettes you smoke.

Light up every other time you have an urge rather than every time, and delay lighting up for as long as possible.

• Make "environmental" changes. Smoke in only one room of your home, and keep cigarettes in an inconvenient place, preferably in another room. Get rid of all but one ashtray, and clean it after each cigarette. Invent your own ways of becoming conscious of every time you want to smoke a cigarette.

Quit. On your chosen day, quit completely. Commit not to smoke. Take things a day at a time, and focus your energy on that one goal. Tomorrow you will take care of tomorrow.

Be aware that you will have difficulties; reflex behavior will have to change when you no longer reach for a cigarette, and nicotine withdrawal may manifest itself as headaches, sleeplessness, irritability, and impatience. You may find it hard to concentrate, and may feel weak, tired, hungry, or depressed. You may cough quite a bit just after quitting. To get through the initial period, you might try the following:

• Change your routine. Have your morning coffee in a chair or room other than the customary one; leave the table immediately after meals; and so on.

• Time your urges by checking your watch when you feel the need for a cigarette. Most urges are short-lived, and realizing this will help you resist.

• Reread the list of reasons why you have committed to quit.

• Accentuate the positive: Drink plenty of water (a full glass every two hours). Use the relaxation techniques described in chapter 4. Communicate through journal writing, and by speaking with your family and support network. If you feel the need, chew sugarless gum or snack on low-calorie foods.

• Avoid the negative: Stay away from situations that provoke the urge for a cigarette, and stay away from smokers whenever possible. When it is not possible, ask them not to light up in front of you.

• Exercise. Physical activity stimulates the production of many of the same endorphins as smoking does. Exercise also stimulates deep breathing, which mimics smoke inhalation, but in a positive, healthy way. And exercise lessens the chance of weight gain.

A study conducted by Dr. Bess Marcus at Brown University examined the effects of exercise in twenty healthy women who were trying to give up smoking. Their program consisted of exercise and/or behavior modification sessions that covered such topics as stress management, relaxation techniques, and coping with cravings and high-risk situations. The quit rate was significantly greater among the women who exercised and took part in the behavior modification than among those in behavior modification alone. By the way, the exercise consisted of only three sessions per week, each lasting thirty to forty-five minutes.

LOW-YIELD TAR AND NICOTINE CIGARETTES

The use of low-yield tar and nicotine cigarettes has *not* been shown to decrease the risk of coronary heart disease. During the last thirty years, the average tar and nicotine yield of American cigarettes has decreased considerably,

and cigarette advertisers have implied that low-yield cigarettes may be safer than conventional ones.

According to the Mayo Clinic, however, low-yield cigarettes contain the same elements as other cigarettes.
These supposedly safer cigarettes have been engineered
simply to make less smoke available to the smoker. Even
filters do not remove carbon monoxide or other harmful
components from tobacco smoke. And since most smokers are addicted to nicotine, when they smoke low-yield
cigarettes they tend to take more frequent puffs and inhale
more deeply. Thus, even after switching to low-yield, they
still may take in at least as much tar, nicotine, and carbon
monoxide as with the older brands.

Approximately 4,000 substances have been identified
in cigarette smoke, including several that are pharmaco-
logically active and toxic. When you consider the presence
of toxic components, and the proven physiological effects
of smoking, and their potential interactions, it is not difficult to understand that low-yield cigarettes are harmful to
your health. The evidence is incontrovertible: Low-yield
cigarettes are not safe. The only safe cigarette is one that
you do not smoke.

Joanne, a patient referred to me, learned the value of
exercise firsthand. A chain-smoking celebrity who lived
near the beach in Malibu, she had been having heart palpitations, which had been worsening over the past year. "I
know you're going to tell me to stop smoking, but forget
it!" she said to me. "Cigarettes are what keep me sane—
from that very first puff in the morning, when I wake up to
the sounds and the smells of that beautiful ocean outside

my door, to the last one at night. Smoking allows me to maintain my sanity." How, I asked her, would she like to appreciate the sounds and the smell of the ocean more than ever *and* deal with her palpitations at the same time. "Oh, really?" she said. "And precisely how do I do that?" "By reaching for your sneakers instead of your cigarettes when you wake up," I said. "If you get into the habit of taking a walk on the beach every morning, you'll feel a hundred percent better than you do now." Months later, Joanne's primary physician told me that Joanne not only was walking on the beach, but also had hired a personal fitness trainer. Moreover—and no surprise—she had stopped smoking and her palpitations had gone away.

Non-Cigarette Nicotine, Hypnotism and Acupuncture, and Support Groups

There are, in addition to the methods suggested above, more structured strategies to quitting.

Most nicotine-addicted smokers have their first cigarette in the first hour after waking in the morning; indeed, many light up even before getting out of bed. Treating this addiction, then, may involve body chemistry as much as behavior modification.

The use of non-cigarette nicotine, together with a program of behavior modification, may be helpful in the early stages of quitting, especially for people who have experienced significant withdrawal symptoms in past attempts to quit. If your first week was extremely difficult, with intense symptoms of craving, uneasiness, and anxiety, you may benefit from nicotine replacement.

Nicotine withdrawal therapy has emerged as a major new means of assisting people to quit smoking. Reports have shown that nicotine withdrawal therapy, *in conjunction with proper counseling and behavior modification, can increase the success rate for quitting over a six-month period.*

Hypnotism and acupuncture each have their strong advocates. The two approaches have similar goals: to use the power of suggestion to increase smokers' confidence that they can do without cigarettes, and to instill positive feelings about the value of what they are doing for themselves. Hypnotized subjects are instructed to play tapes of their sessions whenever they have the urge to smoke, and to gear their thoughts to making cigarettes seem repulsive. The success rates of hypnotism and acupuncture have not been evaluated systematically, but it is clear that they work best when accompanied by a strong belief in them, and when combined with other quit-smoking strategies.

Support groups and clinics have proved more helpful to women than men, from my experience. In general, women are more receptive to these programs and to other participants, and therefore benefit more from them. Men more often prefer going it alone, usually quitting cold turkey.

This was true in my case. I was a second-year medical student smoking one and a half packs a day when I attended a lecture about cigarette smoking given by Dr. Phillip Kersh, a dynamic, charismatic lecturer in pathology. One by one, horrifying images of patients with lung cancer, of black lungs, blocked and occluded arteries, and scarred hearts appeared on the lecture hall screen. They sent audible chills through the hall. The lights went on, and Dr. Kersh paused, took a deep breath, and said, "Every year I give this lecture, and every year a group of you come up to my office, thank me for showing you the truth, take out your pack of cigarettes, put it on my desk, and swear that you're never going to smoke again. Well, if you decide to stop smoking, that's fine. But please do not come to my office and give me your cigarettes, because I will only smoke them myself!" Dr. Kersh, for all his knowledge about the dangers, had continued to smoke. *I*, however, was persuaded; not only did I quit on the spot, but I was able to persuade my parents to quit as well. Dr. Kersh's honest comments at the end of his lecture stayed with me and have helped me understand the enormous difficulties many of my patients have had when trying to quit.

The benefit of a support group can be significant. Such a group offers useful information, a dependable structure, and the opportunity to share experiences—including difficulties—with like-minded people. The contact with people committed to the same goal as yours can strengthen your own resolve. The American Cancer Society and American Lung Association offer stop-smoking clinics, and there are commercial programs available; programs are offered also at many a workplace, and most prove worthwhile. Check with your doctor or local American Cancer Society or Heart or Lung Association branch to find out what is offered in your community.

POTENTIAL PITFALLS

In addition to the difficulties already mentioned in the "Taking Action" section, some women in particular may face the following major obstacles in their attempt to give up smoking:

Concerns about gaining weight. The World Health Organization's recent first international study of tobacco use by women confirmed that women find it more difficult than men to quit smoking, in part because of the fear of gaining weight. The report criticized the tobacco industry for creating "women only" brands and accused it of employing promotional tactics meant to give women the impression that smoking will make them successful, youthful, happy, and slim. "In a weight-conscious, youth-oriented society," says Dr. Karyn Holm, "smoking is thought by many women to be an effective means of weight control, despite knowledge of the hazards of smoking."

It is true that smokers may gain three to five pounds right after quitting. But if you exercise and reduce the fat in your diet when you quit, the weight gain will be minimal and temporary. As a physician, I feel that the obsession that society has placed on women's exterior appearance should never be at the expense of the inner health of your body.

Reliance on smoking as an antidote for unwanted feelings. In the past decade there has been a significant increase in stress levels among women. Many women use cigarettes to cope with stress, as well as anger, fatigue, depression, and other unwanted emotions. Smoking provides a lift, or is calming. By applying the techniques presented in chapter 4 and doing the simple exercise suggested in that chapter, you can learn to deal with your surroundings and your emotions in a healthy way. And this is the path to physical health *and* emotional well-being.

The idea that quitting smoking doesn't seem as important to women as to men. This stems from the myth that smoking is not as serious a health hazard for women as for men. This notion is simply not true. In fact, the Framingham Heart Study showed that a fifty-five-year-old woman who smokes is at *more* risk for a heart attack than a male smoker the same age. It cannot be overemphasized: *If you smoke, quitting is the most important thing you can do for your health.*

GETTING STARTED

Write specific, concrete answers to the following:

1. What is my goal in each "Taking Action" category for the next week?

2. What are my goals for each of the next three weeks after that?

3. When will I start? If not right now, on what day?

4. How will I stick with my plan? What strategies will I use to keep going?

5. What pitfalls may get in my way?

6. What will I do to handle the pitfalls, or avoid them altogether?

7. When will I assess how I am doing with my goals? What will I do to get back on track if I fall short of my goals (join support group, start over)?

RECORDING YOUR PROGRESS

Enter the following in a notebook:

Date
Did I stay with my plan today?
If not, when and how did I go off?
Did any pitfalls come up?
What can I learn from today?

TO SUM UP

1. Fewer women quit smoking than men, and the number of teenage girls who smoke is increasing. This is despite the fact that a fifty-five-year-old woman smoker is in more danger of having a heart attack than a male smoker of the same age.

2. You may lower your health risk substantially if you quit smoking. Your risk of a heart attack decreases within a year after quitting. A recent study found that only three years after quitting, ex-smokers had the same risk of a heart attack as people who never had smoked.

3. It is very difficult for many women to give up smoking, with its deep-seated physical, psychological, and social components. Many smokers are addicted to nicotine, and their habit of turning to cigarettes in many situations has convinced them they cannot cope without smoking.

4. However difficult it may have been, millions of people have kicked the smoking habit. Most who finally manage to quit failed in their initial attempts. Studies show that people who at first fail get better at it with each successive attempt.

5. Your success in quitting depends on two factors: how motivated (and how sick and tired) you are, and how well prepared. Preparation includes weighing your commitment and understanding the tools, strategies, and support you will need to be successful.

6. A solid strategy to stop smoking entails assessing your motivation; understanding withdrawal; considering the use of nicotine replacement or hypnosis, acupuncture, and/or support groups; setting a specific date to quit and informing others.

CHAPTER 9

Mitral Valve Prolapse: The Great Imitator

*Imagination frames events unknown in wild,
fantastic shapes of hideous ruin.*
HANNAH MORE

*There is nothing to fear except the persistent
refusal to find out the truth, the persistent
refusal to analyze the causes of happenings.*
DOROTHY THOMPSON

Michelle, a forty-two-year-old patient of mine, was in a state of severe agitation when I walked into the examination room. Over the last several months, she had become almost incapacitated by recurring bouts of severe chest pains and palpitations, which lasted for hours. She had seen several physicians before coming to me. "They just sat there and told me it was all in my mind," she exclaimed. "That's easy for *them* to say, but these pains and palpitations are real! I've got to get help, or I'm going to lose my mind." I assured Michelle that I knew her symptoms were not imaginary and that we would get to the bottom of her problem.

She was terrified that she was going to have a heart attack, even though it seemed there was no risk of that. Here she was, premenopausal, a nonsmoker, not over-weight—in short, with no risk factors for premature athero-sclerosis. Even more important, her pains had none of the characteristics of angina pectoris—the chest discomfort that suggests the presence of coronary heart disease. When I began the physical exam and listened to Michelle's heart with the stethoscope, the answer was immediately clear. I could hear a distinct clicking sound, followed by a short murmur. The rest of Michelle's exam was completely nor-mal, as was her electrocardiogram. An echocardiogram confirmed a diagnosis of mitral valve prolapse.

Later, we talked about that diagnosis and what it meant. I told Michelle that her problem was not uncom-mon in premenopausal women and that symptoms of se-vere chest pain and palpitations often accompanied mitral valve prolapse. While I would prescribe medication to min-imize the symptoms, she should understand that hers was a benign condition. If she took the medication for a short while, the symptoms would diminish sufficiently to allow a gradual decrease in dosage. I also instructed her to take an antibiotic before any dental work or surgical procedures, to avoid any problem of valve infection.

So she could read more about the disorder, I gave Michelle a pamphlet about mitral valve prolapse provided by the American Heart Association. She was somewhat relieved to know that her problem was real, not imagined, and that something could be done about it. Yet she was still apprehensive. Slowly, over the next month, her symptoms lessened, and her confidence rose accordingly. Six months later, she no longer needed the medication.

Michelle's condition is, as I told her, not uncommon;

mitral valve prolapse—also known as "floppy valve"—occurs particularly in premenopausal women. The term "floppy valve" is quite apt, because during the heart contraction, the valve actually balloons, flops, or "prolapses." By opening and closing in the appropriate timing with the heart contraction, the mitral valve allows the flow of blood in the proper direction from the left atrium to the left ventricle chamber. When the left atrium contracts, the mitral valve opens and blood is propelled into the left ventricle; when the left ventricle contracts, the mitral valve closes and thereby prevents blood from moving back, or regurgitating, into the left atrium. The left ventricle then can pump blood out from the heart to the rest of the body.

Normally, the mitral valve consists of two leaflets, or flaps, shaped like a parachute. They are attached to the heart by cordlike structures known as chordae. Under ordinary circumstances, the valve leaflets close together; but in cases of mitral valve prolapse, when the left ventricle contracts, the mitral valve leaflets do not close evenly. One or both of them balloons or flops back into the left atrium, and a small amount of blood may leak backward through the valve from the left ventricle to the left atrium. The precise reasons for mitral valve prolapse are unknown. It may result from the fact that the valve leaflets are too large or the chords too long (in medical terminology, redundant) or that connective tissue in the valve or chords is more elastic than normal.

Mitral valve prolapse is one of the most prevalent cardiac conditions. Studies reveal that it occurs in as much as 5 to 10 percent of the U.S. population. Since it was first recognized in 1963, it has been diagnosed most frequently in premenopausal women. There has been considerable speculation about its cause, but most current evidence favors a genetic basis for the condition. In various studies, between 20 and 50 percent of the close relatives of people with mitral valve prolapse also had indications of it on their echocardiograms. The majority of these relatives were found to be totally without symptoms. The genetic prevalence seems to be gender-related. In one study, 60 percent of females related to people with mitral valve prolapse had signs of the condition on their echocardiogram, compared with only 27 percent of male relatives. In another, even more striking study, 70 percent of female relatives had echocardiographic evidence of the condition, compared with only 22 percent of male relatives.

The prevalence of mitral valve prolapse increases from childhood to young adulthood, the peak years being between twenty and forty. By the time of menopause, the frequency decreases significantly. While the explanation for this reduction is not clear, the Framingham Heart Study confirmed a steep decline in the occurrence of mitral valve prolapse among older women: from 17 percent of women in their twenties to only 1.4 percent of women in their eighties.

HOW SERIOUS IS MITRAL VALVE PROLAPSE?

The symptoms of mitral valve prolapse are diverse, and they can be frighteningly severe. They often mimic the symptoms of other disorders, such as coronary heart disease, and for this reason I call mitral valve prolapse "the great imitator." It is important to emphasize that for the overwhelming majority of women with the condition, it is neither dangerous nor life-threatening. In fact, recent evidence has shown that the serious consequences and complications of the disorder tend to occur predominantly in men.

Many of the symptoms that accompany mitral valve prolapse may be related to excessive discharges of the nervous system, caused perhaps by stress. Studies have found that some people with the disorder have increased levels of epinephrine and norepinephrine, substances similar to adrenaline, in their bloodstream. Their presence would account for the chest pains, palpitations, shortness of breath, episodes of anxiety, and panic attacks that characterize mitral valve prolapse.

Chest Pain

The reasons for the chest pains of mitral valve prolapse are not totally clear. But it is very clear that no matter how severe and frightening, the pains and other symptoms are *not* dangerous. They will not lead to a heart attack and do not indicate a serious problem. The chest pains of mitral valve prolapse are distinct from, and should be differentiated from, those of angina pectoris; the latter are likely to be due to coronary heart disease and suggest the risk of a heart attack. You should be aware, though, that coronary heart disease and mitral valve prolapse can coexist, and thus the source of pain and other symptoms should be identified.

Barbara, a fifty-four-year-old woman who had been diagnosed several years before as having mitral valve prolapse came to me for further evaluation of chest pains that had been increasing for several weeks. A recent echocardiogram had confirmed the old diagnosis, but when we discussed the nature of her discomfort, it seemed to me there was more going on than just mitral valve prolapse. Barbara described a pressure in the center of her chest that came, for instance, when she walked too fast. When she stopped walking, it went away in a few minutes. The episodes were becoming more frequent and more severe, with less and less physical activity. Barbara already had been to her internist, who prescribed nitroglycerin tablets for her to put under her tongue when she experienced the chest pains, and these had helped significantly.

Barbara had symptoms typical of angina pectoris, namely pressure felt in the center of her chest which was brought on by physical activity and relieved by resting or taking nitroglycerin. Since angina pectoris is usually an indication of coronary heart disease and Barbara's symptoms had increased and become unstable, I recommended a coronary angiogram. Fortunately, the test showed blockage of only one minor coronary artery, and medication helped control her condition.

If you have chest pains that do not match those of angina, and if you are premenopausal, do not smoke, and do not have other risk factors but do have mitral valve prolapse, the chances of your having coronary heart disease are very low. Ordinarily you do not need additional tests, unless of course your physician recommends them. You may find that as your anxiety over the symptoms and diagnosis decreases, so does the severity of the symptoms themselves. Chest pains do go away in most women with mitral valve prolapse.

On the other hand, if your symptoms of chest discomfort suggest angina pectoris or if you are postmenopausal and have additional risk factors (smoking, obesity, diabetes, hypertension, high LDL, or low HDL), it may be wise to be tested for possible coronary heart disease. (See chapter 11 for a discussion of the pluses and minuses of various tests.) Barbara was eight years postmenopausal, and blood tests showed evidence of diabetes with a very low HDL cholesterol level. Key to her diagnosis, however, was the fact that her symptoms were typical of angina pectoris.

The diagnosis of mitral valve prolapse is not difficult, and usually can made by the physician upon listening to the heart with a stethoscope. There is a characteristic "click" in people with mitral valve prolapse, which may be followed by a short heart murmur (as was the case with Michelle). An echocardiogram, a harmless, noninvasive test that accurately visualizes the mitral valve, can confirm the diagnosis.

Heart Murmurs

The significance of a heart murmur is unclear to most people. It is simply a sound, heard when a stethoscope is placed over the heart, caused by turbulence in the bloodstream as it flows through the chambers and valves of the heart. In a sense, the significance of a heart murmur is like the significance of a fever. If you have a fever, it may indicate that you have a harmless virus, but its presence can point also to a more serious infection or other significant illness. Similarly, a heart murmur may be innocent, of no consequence, or it may reflect a potential problem. The most common problems that cause heart murmurs are narrowed or leaky valves. (For a description of the four heart valves, see chapter 10.)

If a murmur is found in someone with mitral valve prolapse, it is usually minor. It simply means that there is a minor leakage of blood from the left ventricle back to the left atrium. This has no serious consequences in the great majority of cases. It does, however, require the precautionary measure of taking antibiotics before and six hours after dental treatment or certain kinds of surgery to prevent possible infection of the valve. In medical procedures such as these, bacteria can enter the bloodstream, and ordinarily the body's defense system removes them. But with a mitral valve leak, bacteria in the blood washing back and forth over the valve may attach themselves to the valve and cause infection (bacterial endocarditis is the medical term).

A small number of people—usually men—with mitral valve prolapse have a heart murmur that indicates more significant mitral regurgitation, or backflow, of blood from the left ventricle to the left atrium. Physical exams, electrocardiograms, and especially echocardiograms are excellent early-detection methods for the few people with more severe mitral valve leaks, so that they can be treated appropriately.

Palpitations

A heart palpitation is an awareness of your heartbeat. It may feel like a pounding, an irregularity, or a skipping in the chest. Like heart murmurs, palpitations can be of no importance. Many people, for example, become aware of their heartbeat during or after vigorous exercise, and this is no cause for alarm. Nor are minor heart rhythm disturbances that are not dangerous in any way. Recurring sensations of rapid, heavy heartbeats or skips should be evaluated. Occasionally the answer will be evident with a routine office electrocardiogram, but since an office ECG records only a few heartbeats, it is often necessary to go further. Stress tests (see chapter 11) and twenty-four-hour ECG monitoring are the most common methods for evaluation. In the latter, the monitor (usually referred to as a Holter), essentially a small ECG machine, is connected to a recording tape that runs for twenty-four hours. Electrodes are put on the patient's chest as in a routine ECG and attached to a recorder placed in a box to be worn over the patient's shoulder. The patient keeps the device on for twenty-four hours while doing normal daily activities. A diary is provided for the patient to record the time of any palpitations, and later the diary is compared with the recording of the heart rhythm to see if there was indeed a significant heart rhythm disturbance at the time the patient felt the palpitations.

Women with mitral valve prolapse frequently have palpitations. The problem is usually minor and requires no medication. On rare occasions, mitral valve prolapse can be associated with a more serious heart rhythm disturbance. This occurs usually among men with characteristic abnormalities signaling high risk on a routine office ECG. These patients often have a severe mitral valve leak as well.

Shortness of Breath, Anxiety, and Panic Attacks

These frightening symptoms often occur together, as was the case with Marilyn, forty-three, who, at the time she came to see me, had reached the point of being afraid to leave her home. For the last few months she had been having sudden attacks of severe shortness of breath, which she described as "so smothering that I absolutely was sure I was going to suffocate." The most recent episode had occurred while Marilyn was standing in line at the supermarket. It was so overwhelming that she started shaking uncontrollably. Finally, she left the line and went to her car, where the symptoms seemingly went on forever.

Marilyn had seen three physicians before coming to my office. "They all thought I was a head case," she told me, "but I know there's something terribly wrong with me."

A physical examination revealed that Marilyn had mitral valve prolapse. There was no valve leak, and her electrocardiogram was normal. I told her that her symptoms were not invented, yet it took a considerable amount of time before she would begin to believe she was not in imminent danger of dying from a heart attack. I prescribed medication to relieve her symptoms, and after a few weeks, Marilyn was able to leave the house for short errands without incident. Slowly and steadily, she managed to resume a normal life. It took several months for her to feel comfortable and confident.

Precisely why Marilyn and other women with mitral valve prolapse experience shortness of breath, anxiety, and panic attacks is not clear. What is known is that these symptoms can be very distressing. Understanding that they can occur with this condition and that, as terrifying as they are, they are not in any way dangerous is a good start to getting them under control. Patience and persistence are crucial here.

PROGNOSIS AND TREATMENT

The outlook for the great majority of people with mitral valve prolapse is excellent. Most will have no symptoms. My experience with patients has been that those women who do have symptoms gradually feel better over time. They come to recognize that their symptoms will not result in a heart attack or worse, and the symptoms themselves thus become less incapacitating. Most women learn to do what Michelle did: "I just put the pains in my handbag and went about my business."

As stated before, the major problem associated with mitral valve prolapse involves a severe leak of blood through the valve, from the left ventricle to the left atrium. Two-thirds of people with such leaks are men, most of them over age fifty. Among women, the main risk with a mitral valve leak's worsening comes if the valve is infected during a dental procedure or certain kinds of surgery. With antibiotics, this risk is preventable. Infections on the mitral valve are, parenthetically, also more likely to occur in men than in women.

Another risk of mitral valve prolapse is a serious heart rhythm disorder. This usually occurs in people who have specific abnormalities on their electrocardiogram (in medical terminology, prolongation of the so-called Q–T interval), and/or severe complex heart rhythm disturbances on the ambulatory twenty-four-hour ECG monitor or during a treadmill exercise test (or both). Severe leakage of the valve is usually present in patients with serious heart rhythm disturbances.

For most women with mitral valve prolapse, treatment focuses on two fronts: preventing infection of the valve, and alleviating severe symptoms. Prophylactic antibiotics are particularly important in fighting infection if there is any leakage across the mitral valve. This can be diagnosed by listening to the heart murmur, or on an echocardiogram. As mentioned above, antibiotics are administered to women with mitral valve prolapse before various types of surgery and dental work. Typically, the patient receives one dosage of the antibiotic an hour or two before the procedure and another dosage six hours later.

Treating the possible symptoms—chest pain, palpitations, shortness of breath, anxiety, panic attacks—begins with realizing that while you may fear their severity, and even fear a heart attack, these symptoms are not dangerous. You will *not* have a heart attack or die. No matter how sick you feel, you *will* be fine; even women with the worst symptoms have an excellent prognosis. And the purpose of medication to treat these symptoms is just that: to alleviate the symptoms, not to protect you from having a heart attack—because you won't be having one.

Medications known as beta blockers (see chapter 11) are available that can decrease the symptoms of mitral valve prolapse significantly. When symptoms become severe, beta blockers can help control them; when symptoms become manageable, the medication can be reduced. Ultimately, even the most severe symptoms abate sufficiently so that medication is no longer needed.

The overwhelming majority of women with mitral valve prolapse can and should live normal, active lives with no restrictions. In fact, a recent study showed that symptoms of the disorder decrease with a regular exercise program. Women who exercised three times a week for twelve weeks had a significant decrease in chest pain, anxiety, and fatigue compared with women who did not exercise.

Even at the risk of sounding repetitive, I must underline the critical psychological factor here: You must keep in mind that your symptoms are not made up in your head and that they do not mean you are having a heart attack or dying. Put your mind at ease. Even if you are diagnosed as having mitral valve prolapse, once this great imitator has been unmasked, you can and will live a normal life.

TO SUM UP

1. Mitral valve prolapse occurs frequently in women between ages twenty and forty; studies have shown that it affects 5 to 10 percent of the U.S. population.

2. Most current evidence points to a genetic basis for the condition.

3. Symptoms accompanying mitral valve prolapse include chest pain, palpitations, shortness of breath, and anxiety and panic attacks. While these symptoms can be severe and frightening, for the overwhelming majority of women, mitral valve prolapse is not life-threatening.

4. The major problems associated with mitral valve prolapse are significant leakage across the mitral valve and serious heart rhythm disorder. These problems occur primarily in men over age fifty and are diagnosed by finding specific abnormalities on echocardiograms and electrocardiograms.

5. The treatment for most women with mitral valve prolapse is twofold: preventing infection on the mitral valve by using prophylactic antibiotics before dental work or certain types of surgery, and treating the symptoms when they are severe.

CHAPTER 10

How Your Heart Works, in Health and Disease

*Oh, wondrous power! How little understood
. . . to fashion genius, form the soul for good.*
SARAH J. HALE

*Knowledge . . . should sharpen our ability to
scrutinize more steadily.*
MARGARET MEAD

Your heart is a beautifully designed pump whose purpose is to deliver blood, together with life-giving oxygen and nutrients, to every cell, tissue, and organ of your body. Shaped something like a pear, and weighing about eleven ounces, the heart sits in the center of the chest, pointing up toward the right shoulder. It is a specialized muscle divided into four chambers, two on the right and two on the left, which are separated by one-way valves. The heart therefore is in a sense two pumps, because its right and left sides are separated from each other.

CIRCULATION

There are four chambers in the heart, two—an atrium and a ventricle—on either side. The right atrium is a receptacle for the veins transporting blood back into the heart. It receives blood from the veins after it has traveled through the body and given the tissues their needed allotment of oxygen and nutrients. When the right atrium has filled, it contracts and pushes its contents through the tricuspid valve and into the right ventricle.

The right ventricle transports oxygen-depleted blood to the lungs. When the chamber contracts, it moves its contents across the pulmonary valve into the pulmonary artery and its branches in the lungs. The blood travels into progressively smaller arteries, and eventually into tiny vessels called capillaries. These blood vessels have very thin and delicate linings that allow oxygen and other nutrients to move into and out of the bloodstream. While in the capillaries, the blood and its red blood cells come into contact with alveoli, small air sacs filled with the oxygen-rich air taken in with each breath. The oxygen in the alveoli moves across the capillary membrane and into the blood, where it joins with the red cells. The bloodstream not only picks up oxygen but also eliminates carbon dioxide waste products, received from the tissues and cells of the body, to the lung air sacs. From the lungs, the carbon dioxide can be exhaled into the atmosphere.

Once these exchanges have been completed, the blood moves through the pulmonary capillaries into the pulmonary veins for delivery to the left side of the heart. The left atrium is the collecting chamber for blood returning to the heart from the lungs. Once it is full, the left atrium contracts and moves its contents across the mitral valve and into the left ventricle.

The left ventricle is by far the most powerful pumping chamber of the heart. Its contents must be propelled under pressure much higher than in the other chambers, so that the oxygen-enriched blood can travel through the arteries of the entire body at a sufficient pressure to reach every cell and organ. As the left ventricle receives blood, it tenses and builds energy which is released with a powerful contraction that sends the blood through the aortic valve and into the aorta, the largest artery in the body. From there the blood continues flowing to the major arteries and on to the rest of the body. The artery networks get progressively smaller, ending finally in a microscopic network of capillaries.

Oxygen and nutrients in the blood now can diffuse through the delicate membranes of these capillaries, resupplying its designated area. Waste products from these cells and tissues are transported into the bloodstream, to be carried to three main waste dumps—the lungs, kidneys, and liver—and then expelled from the body. When these transactions have been completed, the blood moves on from the capillaries to the veins for transportation back to the right atrium of the heart. The cycle is complete, and begins anew.

This extraordinary round-trip takes about a minute and repeats itself every minute of your life. In an average person's lifetime, it is estimated, the heart contracts 2.5 billion times. Each day, the average heart beats some 100,000 times and pumps more than 2,000 gallons' worth of blood through the equivalent of approximately 60,000 miles of blood vessels.

THE HEART VALVES

The heart valves serve an important function, ensuring that the flow of blood continues in a one-way direction from the right side of the heart, through the lungs, to the left side of the heart, and then to the rest of the body. When the right atrium contracts, for example, the tricuspid valve opens, allowing blood into the right ventricle. When the right ventricle contracts, the pulmonary valve opens, allowing blood into the blood vessels of the lungs, at the same time the tricuspid valve shuts. This simultaneous action prevents the blood in the right ventricle from moving backward into the right atrium.

Similarly, on the left side of the heart, when the left atrium contracts, the mitral valve opens, allowing blood into the left ventricle. When it contracts, the aortic valve opens, allowing blood from the left ventricle into the aorta and other arteries. At the same moment, the mitral valve snaps shut, preventing any backflow of blood from the left ventricle to the left atrium. When the left ventricle completes its contraction and relaxes, the pressure in it falls, and the pressure in the aorta is then higher than in the left ventricle. But when the aortic valve snaps shut, it prevents the blood in the aorta from returning, or regurgitating, into the left ventricle.

The valves themselves are delicate structures, connected by chords to strong rings at their base. Abnormalities of the heart valves can be due to a variety of conditions (most commonly infections and diseases, such as rheumatic fever, and congenital defects). These disorders may cause the valves to develop leaks or become narrowed, or both. The mitral and aortic valves, on the left side of the heart, are more prone to these abnormalities than the right-side tricuspid and pulmonary valves. A valve leak or backflow is referred to as regurgitation; a valve narrowing is known as stenosis.

HEART FAILURE

When a heart valve is badly damaged and the leak and/or narrowing severe, it can put sufficient strain on the heart to cause dysfunction and the condition known as heart failure. The heart's output to the body becomes reduced because it is working under prolonged stress. To compensate for the stress, the heart enlarges. When this no longer can overcome the continuing strain of overwork, fluid from the bloodstream begins to back up into the lungs. This results in symptoms of progressive shortness of breath. Patients can have difficulty breathing during physical activity or when lying flat (and they must prop themselves up with pillows to sleep). Swelling, or edema, of the feet and ankles can also develop.

Heart failure can occur not only as a result of valvular disease but also because of hypertension, coronary heart disease, and heart muscle disorders. With hypertension, high pressure in the arteries forces the heart, specifically the left ventricle, to pump against very high resistance. The left ventricle attempts to compensate for this with an increase in muscle mass. When this enlargement, called hypertrophy, no longer suffices, heart failure develops. With coronary heart disease, heart failure results when the amount of damage to the left ventricle, the most vulnerable chamber for a heart attack, exceeds 40 percent of the total muscle. The amount of functioning heart muscle remaining is then inadequate to meet the needs of the body.

Heart muscle disorders, or cardiomyopathies, are due to a number of conditions. The most common are viral infections, in which case a virus attacks the heart muscle, and excessive consumption of alcohol, which acts as a heart muscle poison in some people. When the heart muscle has been weakened too much, heart failure is the consequence.

BLOOD PRESSURE AND HEARTBEAT

Blood pressure is the tension of the blood against the walls of the arteries. The walls of the arteries are elastic, and they stretch when blood is propelled into them under pressure. In a blood pressure reading, the top number indicates the systolic pressure, the pressure generated on the arteries by the blood when it is ejected by the left ventricle during its contraction. If the artery walls are stiff, systolic pressure (and the top number in a blood pressure reading) is elevated. The bottom number, representing diastolic pressure, indicates the tension and resistance on the artery walls while the heart is resting between contractions, since this pressure is measured when the left ventricle relaxes. Normal blood pressure is 120/80; high blood pressure, or hypertension, is usually defined as a reading above 140/90 on three consistent occasions, but it may be an elevation of either systolic or diastolic pressure alone as well. Untreated hypertension causes excessive stress on the arteries and can lead to heart attack, stroke, heart failure, or kidney disease (see chapter 7 for more details).

The heartbeat is brought about by an electrical discharge from an area of specialized heart muscle called the sinoatrial node. Located high in the right atrium, this tissue regularly sends a wavelike impulse down the right and left atria. The impulse reaches a second node, the atrioventricular node, pauses briefly, and then continues through specialized heart muscle across the right and left ventricles. The right and left atria contract simultaneously and empty their contents (blood) into the two corresponding ventricles. The right ventricle then contracts and empties its contents into the pulmonary artery, while the left ventricle similarly propels its contents into the aorta. The heart's electrical activity can be recorded with an electrocardiogram, which can detect heart rhythm disturbances as well as other abnormalities (see chapter 11).

THE CORONARY ARTERIES AND ATHEROSCLEROSIS

Like the other organs of the body, the hardworking heart requires oxygen and nutrients to function. This need is served by the coronary arteries, two small vessels on the outer surface of the heart, both of which originate from the aorta, just above the aortic valve. The right coronary artery supplies the undersurface of the heart. The left coronary artery runs for about an inch at the top of the heart before it divides into two main branches called the left anterior descending, going to the front of the heart, and circumflex, supplying the back of the heart. These three arteries (right, left anterior descending, and circumflex) and their branches send smaller tributaries into the substance of the heart muscle which supply it with the oxygen and nutrients needed to contract and pump normally.

The coronary arteries are more susceptible than most of the other arteries of the body to atherosclerosis, a buildup of cholesterol within artery walls. If great enough, this buildup may obstruct the artery. Under resting conditions, the blood flowing through the diseased coronary artery may be sufficient to supply a specific area of heart muscle, but under more demanding conditions such as exercise, when the heart is working harder and requires more oxygen and nutrients, the obstruction may not allow sufficient blood through to meet the needs of the heart area it supplies. What is created, then, is an imbalance of oxygen supply and demand. When a significant area of heart muscle is in this state (known in medicine as ischemia), the individual affected usually experiences symptoms of chest discomfort called angina pectoris.

Angina pectoris is the first sign of coronary artery disease in women: 56 percent have anginal chest pain as their initial coronary disease problem, compared with 43 percent of men. When angina begins in women, it is usually stable; it occurs predictably during physical activity and is relieved promptly with rest. When you are at rest, your heart is working less hard and requires less oxygen, and even an obstructed coronary artery remains capable of maintaining adequate blood supply.

However, a diseased artery can become progressively more obstructed and unstable. A disruption or tear in the inner lining of the artery usually indicates urgent problems. The artery can go into spasm, the blood flow through it decreasing further and thus critically reducing the supply of oxygen to the heart muscle, even though the affected individual may not be engaging in physical activity. (Angina that occurs with an individual at rest is referred to as unstable angina.) More important, the disrupted portion of the coronary artery is now prone to thrombosis, or clotting, on its inner surface, which also can further reduce the oxygen supply.

Symptoms of unstable angina usually can be relieved with nitroglycerin, but they need to be taken seriously, because they may be the warning signs of an impending heart attack. When a clot completely obstructs, or occludes, a diseased coronary artery, the portion of heart muscle supplied by that artery becomes starved for vital oxygen and nutrients. If the occlusion persists for more than one hour, the affected heart muscle begins to die. This is usually accompanied by severe, persistent crushing pain over the center of the chest, the prime symptom of a heart attack.

About one-third of women with coronary heart disease have a heart attack as the first evidence of the problem, compared with half of men. However, initial heart attacks are more likely to be fatal in women (39 percent versus 31 percent for men). In the Framingham Heart Study, 68 percent of all coronary heart disease deaths in women occurred during the first heart attack, compared with 49 percent for men. Women also have an increased occurrence of heart attacks that go unrecognized, 35 percent versus 27 percent for men. Further in the Framingham study, the rate of death within one year after a heart attack was 45 percent for women, in contrast to 10 percent for men. Stroke was also more common in women after a heart attack, 12.7 percent versus 7.7 percent in men. These statistics provide compelling evidence that preventing heart attack is a crucial goal for women at risk.

Medications are now available that can break up and dissolve blood clots responsible for a heart attack. If these "clot busters," or thrombolytics, are given within the first few hours of a heart attack, the clot usually can be dissolved and blood flow through the coronary artery can be restored, and at least a portion of the dying heart muscle can be salvaged. The amount of heart muscle saved depends primarily on the duration of the heart attack and the promptness with which the medication is given. Clot busters administered within the first few hours of a heart attack have been shown to decrease the risk of mortality.

Most people who reach the hospital survive heart attacks and can live normal lives afterward. The heart is a remarkably resilient organ. It can suffer significant damage before impairment in function occurs. The outlook for patients with coronary heart disease depends on the extent of blockage in the major coronary arteries and the extent of heart muscle damage from the heart attack. It is important for anyone who has angina pectoris or who has recovered from a heart attack to undergo a careful evaluation of his or her condition, as the next chapter will discuss.

CHAPTER 11

Heart Disease: Tests and Treatments

*We are solely responsible for our choices and
we have to accept the consequences.*
ELISABETH KÜBLER-ROSS

*Heed the still, small voice that so seldom leads
us wrong and never into folly.*
MADAME DU DEFFAND

The number of available tests and treatments for heart
problems may seem bewildering and intimidating. Applied
properly, they can be enormously helpful in clarifying
problems and dealing effectively with them. To facilitate
the task of sorting out your options, keep in mind these
basic principles of testing and treatment:

• The purpose of any test is twofold: first, to assist in
making an accurate diagnosis, if it is not already clear; and
second, to assess the severity of a problem, particularly if

important changes in treatment are being considered, such as heart surgery or coronary angioplasty.

• The goals of treatment are threefold: first, to prolong your life if possible; second, to prevent a heart attack (if your potential problem is coronary heart disease); and third, to alleviate symptoms and thereby to improve the quality of your life.

• For optimal diagnosis and therapy, good communication between patient and doctor is essential. This means that you understand your situation, as well as the benefits and risks of a recommended test or treatment. (See "Communicating with Your Doctor About Tests" and "Communicating with Your Doctor About Therapy" on pages 161 and 173.)

This chapter will discuss the fundamentals of the major tests and treatments for heart problems. It begins with the most basic and proceeds to the more complex.

TESTS

Electrocardiogram

An electrocardiogram, or ECG or EKG, records the various peaks and valleys of the heart's electrical activity and the spread of impulses from the atrial to the ventricular chambers. The electrocardiogram has long been invaluable for detecting cardiac abnormalities. It can record heart rhythm disturbances, or arrhythmias, and assess their severity, risk, and need for therapy. If you have palpitations, or if there is a suspicion that heart rhythm disturbances may be present that do not appear on an office ECG, a recording can be made of your heart rhythm over a twenty-four-hour period. See page 144 for a description of this daylong Holter monitoring.

Some cardiologists advocate using the Holter monitor to detect silent ischemia, an imbalance which is created by an inadequate supply of oxygen to the heart because of an obstructed coronary artery and which does not show the usual symptoms of anginal chest discomfort. I do not recommend the Holter for this purpose, as the evidence for its usefulness has not convinced me.

COMMUNICATING WITH YOUR DOCTOR ABOUT TESTS

Communication with your physician is always important, especially if he or she is recommending tests for you. Asking your doctor the following questions may help you gain a better understanding of your situation.

• What is the purpose of the test? What will it indicate? Will it clarify the diagnosis, assess the severity of the problem, guide therapy, or do otherwise?

• How likely is it (what are the percentage chances) that the test will accomplish this purpose? What is the percentage of accuracy of the test in your specific situation?

• How is the test performed?

• What kind of preparation is necessary?

• What risks are involved, and what is their likelihood?

• Will the test be painful?

• What is the recovery time?

• Is the test absolutely necessary?

- When will the results be known?
- Will the results give a clear answer, or will additional tests be necessary?

It is also appropriate to ask about a test *you* think may be helpful, if questions about your diagnosis or treatment do not seem fully answered.

- Would an additional test provide useful information about my condition? If not, why not?
- Could there be value in doing:

A nuclear heart scan, to clarify my chest pain?
A Holter monitor test, to clarify my palpitations?
A chest X ray, to clarify my shortness of breath?
An echocardiogram, to clarify my murmur?
An echocardiogram, to clarify my mitral valve prolapse?
If not, why not?

When discussing tests or treatments with your doctor, it can be helpful to bring along a friend or family member. Take paper and pen to write down the important points of the conversation, to minimize confusing the details later.

═══

The electrocardiogram can provide other information, about heart muscle damage from a heart attack and heart chamber enlargement, for instance. However, the ECG is not sensitive enough to pick up all significant heart problems. Abnormalities can exist without appearing on the electrocardiogram, and other tests may be necessary to explore their presence and severity. A routine office ECG, for example, taken as you rest on an examination table, is not very useful if you have angina pectoris. Your heart needs to be stressed for characteristic abnormalities to be seen. An ECG also is not as accurate as an echocardiogram (see below) in detecting enlargement of the heart chambers.

Besides giving normal readings in the presence of heart disease, an ECG may give false readings of abnormality in people without heart disease. This simple office test, then, is at best a screen for *some* cases of heart disease; ECG readings must be interpreted in the context of other evidence, such as a patient's medical history and physical exam.

Chest X Ray

The chest X ray, like the electrocardiogram, has long been a routine part of an initial cardiac evaluation. Its major purpose is to evaluate the size of the heart chambers and aorta, as well as the state of the lungs. While enlargement of the heart chambers is visible on an X ray, an echocardiogram (see below) is a more sensitive way to detect it. The chest X ray is very useful for detecting pulmonary abnormalities and is important in indicating the presence of fluid in the lungs as a result of heart failure (see chapter 9). When the heart chambers and valves need to be evaluated more accurately—in, say, a patient with a heart murmur—an echocardiogram is a more accurate test.

Echocardiogram

This test, painless, harmless, and easily performed, uses ultrasonic waves to evaluate the chambers and valves of the heart. When the ultrasound is reflected back from the chest to the recording device, accurate and valuable information is obtained about the size of the four heart chambers and the presence of valvular disease. Abnormalities in heart contraction can also be detected.

The echocardiogram is often used in conjunction with the Doppler study, which evaluates the speed of the blood as it passes through the valves from one heart chamber to the next. By accurately sensing turbulent blood flow patterns, the Doppler helps in diagnosing narrowed and/or leaking heart valves and evaluating heart murmurs. Important information about the severity of valve abnormalities and their effect on the heart chambers can be gathered from this combination of echocardiogram and Doppler study.

An echocardiogram was especially helpful in diagnosing a thirty-eight-year-old patient, Paula, for whom electrocardiogram and chest X ray had proved inadequate. Paula was sent to me because she had become progressively short of breath and fatigued over a six-month period. "I've reached a point where I can't walk one full block without gasping for air. I feel exhausted all the time," she told me. The records Paula brought with her indicated a normal heart exam. Both her electrocardiogram and her X ray could have been read as normal. When I listened closely to Paula's heart, there was a faint murmur, but I couldn't be certain about the diagnosis.

An echocardiogram showed clearly that Paula's heart chambers were enlarged and the heart's contractions weakened. She suffered from cardiomyopathy, a disorder of the heart muscle which decreases its ability to contract normally. Her heart valves were normal. We gave Paula medication, and her symptoms improved.

Stress Test (Treadmill Exercise ECG)

The stress test is a reasonably safe way to assess chest pains that suggest the possibility of coronary heart disease. In patients who recently have suffered a heart attack, it is used to predict the risk of another. Stress tests, as previously discussed, are used to screen middle-aged men and women for specific purposes—such as approval for a vigorous exercise program—and to unmask heart rhythm disturbances. The patient, walking on a treadmill, is hooked up to an ECG and wears a blood pressure cuff; the heart is made to increase its workload gradually, as the speed and slope of the treadmill increase. The heart rate increases, and likewise the heart's need of oxygen. If any of the coronary arteries is obstructed, a critical level is reached in which the supply of blood and oxygen to the heart muscle can no longer keep up with the increasing demand. Under these circumstances, a patient may begin to experience symptoms of angina pectoris and characteristic changes, known as ST segment depression, may develop on the electrocardiogram.

If there are no changes in the ECG, the patient continues walking on the treadmill until the heart rate reaches a predetermined maximum. (This target rate, as mentioned earlier, is calculated by subtracting the patient's age from 220.) Many cardiologists prefer "submaximal" stress tests, at 70 to 90 percent of the maximum heart rate, for greater safety. These lower rates lessen the possibility of severe anginal symptoms, severe new abnormalities suggesting coronary blockage, severe heart rhythm abnormalities, and severe shortness of breath or fatigue in the patient.

If the changes characteristic of coronary heart disease

manifest themselves on the ECG, the test is called positive. The accuracy of a positive test is higher if:

- Anginal chest discomfort develops during the test.
- The ST segment depression occurs early in the test and at a low heart rate.
- The amount of ST segment depression is substantial.
- Blood pressure decreases during the test.

Note, however, the possibility of false positive and false negative tests: A patient can have a positive stress test and not have coronary heart disease. Conversely, a patient can have a normal stress test and still have coronary heart disease. The incidence of both false positive and false negative tests is notoriously high in women.

While the stress test can be useful in assessing women who recently have recovered from a heart attack, and as a screen, its accuracy for women is low. In addition, all stress tests are dangerous when unstable symptoms are present. If you have had anginal symptoms that occurred only with exercise and now are occurring with exercise and at rest, a stress test should not be done, because of the risk of precipitating a heart attack. In general, then, I believe a nuclear heart scan is the best method for evaluating suspicious chest discomfort that suggests coronary heart disease in women.

Nuclear Heart Scans

A nuclear heart scan is the best initial means of diagnosing coronary heart disease in women with suspicious chest pain. It is performed identically to the stress test after which a small amount of a radioactive substance called thallium (or a similar isotope) is injected into a vein. The isotope gets taken up by the heart muscle while a recording of its distribution is made with a gamma camera. The patient is asked to return several hours later for a "rest scan" to compare with the "exercise scan."

Norma, forty-eight years old, came to me for an evaluation after a positive stress test. Naturally, she was nervous that she might have a coronary heart disease problem, even though she had no symptoms and the stress test had been done as part of a routine checkup. Apart from a slightly elevated cholesterol of 210, Norma had no risk factors for heart disease. But in view of the positive stress ECG, I felt a nuclear heart scan should be done to clarify the situation. It proved to be normal, and I was able to assure Norma that she was fine and would need no further testing.

Two conditions are required for the isotope to be distributed normally by the heart: the coronary arteries must be open to deliver it, and the heart muscle must not have any severe scarring from a previous heart attack, since scar tissue cannot absorb the thallium or isotope. During the exercise scan, if a "cold spot" is observed—that is, the substance is not detected by the gamma camera—there is either a blockage of the coronary artery to that area of the heart or a scar from a previous heart attack is preventing uptake of the isotope. If the cold spot disappears during the rest scan, the heart muscle is normal (if it were scarred, the scan would remain cold) and the abnormality detected in the exercise scan is due to a blocked coronary artery. If the cold spot persists, it strongly suggests a scarred area. These findings are called "reversible" and "irreversible" defects.

Patients who cannot exercise adequately can undergo other methods of stressing the heart. Frequently a drug is given intravenously to stress the heart; the most popular currently is dipyridamole. After the desired effect on the heart has been produced, the thallium or isotope is injected and its distribution recorded.

The nuclear heart scan is a very useful test for diagnosing coronary heart disease in women who have been having suspicious chest pain or who have a positive stress test but no symptoms. Its risks are minor and identical to those of the stress ECG. As with any stress test, a nuclear scan should not be performed on someone who is having unstable anginal symptoms.

Cardiac Catheterization and Coronary Arteriography

Cardiac catheterization is a procedure in which the pressures in the heart chambers and across the valves are measured as well as the function of the heart. Coronary arteriography is the process in which contrast dye is injected into the coronary arteries while a continuous X ray is taken. The dye allows the coronary arteries to be seen in great detail, thus providing an accurate road map of the vessels. The presence, location, severity, and number of obstructions can be visualized accurately on the X-ray film recording, and the cardiologist can determine whether there is a coronary artery problem, how serious it is, and what, if anything, need be done (e.g., bypass surgery or angioplasty, discussed later in this chapter). In a procedure known as ventriculography, dye can be injected into the left ventricle to assess its pumping ability and the presence of any contraction abnormalities. Normally, cardiac catheterization and coronary arteriography are performed at the same time, and the two terms often are used interchangeably.

These procedures are by far the most accurate way to evaluate the heart and the coronary arteries. They are not, however, appropriate for everyone with a possible heart problem. The studies are invasive, requiring a physician to insert long, thin tubes (catheters, hence the name of the procedure) into the blood vessels of the groin or arm, from where they are advanced, with an X ray for guidance, to the heart. This entails a small risk and some discomfort, and requires your going to the hospital.

While cardiac catheterization and coronary arteriography are the most accurate tests, they should be performed only under certain circumstances. First, if a serious problem is still suspected after previous tests have been inconclusive—when, for instance, a woman has severe chest pain thought to be angina and her nuclear heart scan is equivocal. Second, if a problem is deemed severe enough that it might require further intervention such as bypass surgery or angioplasty—when, for instance, a woman with angina is stable but her nuclear heart scan suggests severe disease. And third, if there is a high likelihood of unstable angina; a stress test or nuclear heart scan is riskier than arteriography under these circumstances, and the arteriogram will show quickly whether or not bypass surgery or angioplasty is needed.

Which Test, and Under What Circumstances?

The following examples may give you a better understanding of what test or tests might be done in a particular situation. Discussing your alternatives with your doctor is the key to making good choices. (See the sections "Communicating with Your Doctor About Tests" and "Communicating with Your Doctor About Therapy" on pages 161 and 173.)

If you have chest pain, the most important way to tell whether it is due to coronary heart disease is whether or not the discomfort is characteristic of angina pectoris. If your symptoms are those of typical angina—pressure sensation in the center of the chest which is brought on by physical exertion and relieved by rest—the probabilities are high that you have coronary heart disease. If your chest discomfort feels like the pressure sensation of angina, but is not brought on by physical activity, you are experiencing atypical angina. In this case, the chance that you have coronary artery disease is about one in three, or 30 to 40 percent. And if you are feeling nonspecific chest pain, chest discomfort with none of the characteristics of angina, the chance that you have coronary artery disease is at most one in twenty.

If you have definite or probable angina, I recommend a stress test or a nuclear heart scan. If the test or scan is normal, the likelihood is high that you do not have coronary heart disease or that the problem is minor. Usually there is no reason to go further, that is, to have coronary arteriography or any other procedure. If, on the other hand, the stress test or nuclear scan suggests coronary heart disease *and* significant blockage in more than one of the major arteries, coronary arteriography may be necessary. It will locate the blockages precisely, and indicate whether bypass surgery or angioplasty is needed.

If you have a heart murmur which may be caused by a valve narrowing or leak, the most useful test is an echocardiogram in conjunction with a Doppler study. Valvular problems can be detected quite accurately. It also provides valuable information about their effect on the heart chambers and a reasonable estimate of the severity of the problem. If your symptoms, physical exam, and echocardiogram suggest a severe valvular disorder and heart dysfunction, cardiac catheterization is needed to assess the situation more fully and accurately and to determine whether valve surgery is necessary.

RECOVERING FROM A HEART ATTACK

If you have recovered recently from a heart attack, you should be evaluated to determine whether or not there is another immediate threat, i.e., a second severely blocked coronary artery that could occlude, causing another heart attack. In these circumstances, a stress electrocardiogram (which is more accurate in these circumstances for women than as a diagnostic test for chest pain) or a nuclear heart scan is useful. If the test shows the possibility of an additional problem, coronary arteriography can be done to assess the situation further. However, if the test is negative, I would encourage you to enter a cardiac rehabilitation program.

A heart attack is a frightening experience, and understandably, many people remain fearful and depressed after they leave the hospital. You need as much support as possible after a heart attack. Studies have shown that a solid support system of family and friends significantly improves recovery.

A cardiac rehabilitation program provides additional support. Being with people who have gone through the same experience helps decrease feelings of isolation. Cardiac rehabilitation programs can be wonderfully upbeat, with a contagious optimism. You are engaged in specific activities designed to restore you to a normal life and lessen the likelihood of future heart attacks. The hands-on guidance you receive will increase your confidence and speed your return to good health.

TREATMENTS

As I have said before, you need to understand your own problem fully, and its treatment as well. Keep in mind the specific goals of any recommended treatment: to prolong your life if possible; to prevent a heart attack; and to improve the quality of your life by decreasing the frequency and severity of your symptoms.

Coronary Bypass Surgery

This type of surgery entails the insertion of a vein (usually the saphenous vein, from the leg) or an artery (usually the mammary artery, from the chest wall), so as to reroute the flow of blood around a blocked coronary artery. By thus "bypassing" the blockage, normal delivery of blood and oxygen to an otherwise jeopardized area of heart muscle can occur. When a vein is used (specifically, the saphenous vein), it is sutured into the aorta on one end and into the diseased coronary artery, "downstream" from the area of blockage, on the other. When an artery is used (specifically, the mammary artery), it is lifted from the chest wall and implanted into the coronary artery past the blockage.

COMMUNICATING WITH YOUR DOCTOR ABOUT THERAPY

It is important that you understand any treatment recommended by your doctor. If anything is unclear, asking the following questions may be useful.

• What is the purpose of the treatment? Is it to prolong life, to prevent eventual disease, to decrease symptoms, or otherwise?

• How likely is it (what are the percentage chances) that the treatment will accomplish this goal?

• As far as surgery or angioplasty is concerned:
What are the percentage chances of my making it through the operation?
What are the chances of complications? What are they? How serious are they?
How much pain and discomfort may be involved?
How much time is involved, in the hospital, in rehabilitation, before returning to normal activities?

• What are the alternatives? What are their comparative risks and benefits? What are the advantages of a more conservative or a more aggressive approach?

Bypass surgery can be a wonderful, lifesaving operation. It can prolong the life of people with severe blockages of all three major coronary arteries (or a blockage in the left main coronary artery) and previous heart muscle damage. In particular, it has been a dramatic answer for patients with unstable anginal chest pains and severe diffuse blockages.

However, the bypass should not be done indiscriminately. If the blockages are less widespread, a more conservative approach is warranted.

Despite troubling statistics that indicate a higher risk with bypass surgery among women than among men, I feel it is still a good choice for some women. If you have severe or unstable symptoms of angina pectoris and show evidence of serious, widespread blockage, a bypass should be considered. Relying on medication in these critical circumstances is riskier than the operation, and your chances of living long afterward are better with the bypass.

Coronary Angioplasty

Several forms of coronary angioplasty are being used currently to relieve blockages in these arteries. In the most common procedure, a long, thin tube with a tiny deflated balloon on the end is introduced into a blocked coronary artery. The balloon is positioned in the area of the blockage and inflated. The artery in the diseased area is thus dilated, and the atherosclerotic material is pushed against the artery wall. The tube, with its balloon, is withdrawn from the artery, now dilated so that normal blood flow is restored. Other forms of relieving coronary blockage include *laser angioplasty*, in which a laser on the end of the tube is used to vaporize the blockage, and *atherectomy*, in which the atherosclerotic material is removed through the catheter.

Like coronary bypass surgery, angioplasty is somewhat less effective for women than for men: with women patients there is lower initial success in opening the blocked artery, as well as more complications and a higher risk. The long-term results, however, are favorable among women.

After successful angioplasty, most women see substantial improvement in their symptoms and have an excellent outlook. Angioplasty involves much less discomfort than does bypass surgery, and a relatively short hospitalization and rehabilitation period. It is common for more than one blocked coronary artery to be dilated per procedure.

A big problem with angioplasty is the recurrence of coronary blockage. Reclosing occurs in more than 30 percent of vessels that have been opened, and the rate is closer to 40 percent in patients who were unstable at the time of the procedure. This is true for the balloon, laser, and atherectomy procedures. Most reclosures come early—as soon as three to six months after the procedure—and patients usually experience anginal symptoms again and may require a second dilation. Unfortunately, blockage is frequent after a second angioplasty as well. Nonetheless, I recommend angioplasty for women with severe or unstable angina and one or two blocked coronary arteries, because the results are usually better than with medications alone.

MEDICATIONS

Various drugs are available that may not only minimize your symptoms and make you feel better, but also decrease your risk of heart problems. Some of them are described below.

Anti-anginal Medications

Anti-anginal drugs are meant to correct any imbalance between the amount of blood, including oxygen, being delivered to the heart muscle and the amount of oxygen the heart muscle requires. Three categories of drugs have proved effective in the treatment of anginal symptoms: nitrates, beta blockers, and calcium channel blockers.

Nitrates. By dilating the blood vessels, these agents allow an increase in blood flow through a blocked coronary artery to the heart. Their primary benefit, however, is in dilating the arteries of the body so that the heart can work less hard to pump blood, and thus require less oxygen to do its job. The balance between oxygen supply and demand is improved, and anginal symptoms decrease.

There are several types of nitrate preparations. Nitroglycerin, in the form of tablets placed under the tongue, is used to control an episode of anginal symptoms as it occurs, or is employed as a prophylactic before a walk, sex, or any activity that might cause anginal symptoms. Its effect begins in minutes and lasts up to an hour. Among the longer-acting nitrate preparations that can reduce the frequency and severity of anginal symptoms are oral medicines such as *isosorbide dinitrate* and *mononitrate*, whose effects last for three to four hours, and *transdermal nitroglycerin patches*, which are put on the upper arms or back.

Nitrates, which have been in use for more than a century, are quite safe; side effects are rare and, when they occur, usually are not serious. The most common is headache, but this normally disappears after the medication has been used for a week or two. Other possible side effects are dizziness, weakness, upset stomach, and skin rash, and all disappear when the medication is stopped.

Beta blockers. These agents lower the amount of oxygen the heart muscle needs by slowing it down and reducing the force with which it contracts. This substantially eases the workload of the heart and decreases the symptoms of angina pectoris.

Beta blockers often are prescribed for conditions other than angina pectoris. They are effective in treating hypertension and certain heart rhythm disturbances, and have been recommended for some patients recovering from a heart attack, to reduce the risk of another attack or sudden death.

In general, beta blockers are well tolerated and side effects are minor. However, they all have potential side effects. Beta blockers should *not* be taken by patients with lung diseases such as emphysema or asthma, since they can worsen these conditions; likewise for patients with heart failure, since beta blockers weaken the contraction of the heart. Among other possible side effects are excessively reduced heart rate, fatigue, mental depression, cold sensation in the extremities, hair loss, and skin rash.

Calcium channel blockers. These drugs are the most recently developed agents for treating angina, and they are very effective. Like nitrates, they are powerful dilators of blood vessels and increase blood flow through the coronary arteries, particularly in patients with some degree of spasm in these blood vessels. By dilating arteries in the body, calcium channel blockers allow the heart to work less hard to pump blood. Like beta blockers, they decrease the force of the heart's contraction somewhat, and thus its oxygen requirements.

Calcium channel blockers are important drugs used in the treatment of angina and hypertension. There are several available, and side effects differ among them.

For Prevention: Aspirin and Cholesterol-Lowering Drugs

ASPIRIN

Simple aspirin has come to play an important role in the treatment of coronary heart disease. It is an antiplatelet drug, one of a group of medications that keep clotting elements in the blood called platelets from sticking to each other and to the walls of the arteries. When the lining of a coronary artery is injured, if the blood platelets are less able to stick to the damaged area and form a clot, there is less chance of heart attack.

Several studies have shown that taking one baby aspirin daily reduces the risk of a second heart attack in patients who have recovered from their first. Aspirin has proved helpful also in preventing strokes and keeping grafts open in patients who have had coronary bypass surgery.

The primary side effects of aspirin are upset stomach and a tendency to bleed. Occasionally it can cause allergic reaction or skin rash.

CHOLESTEROL-LOWERING DRUGS

If a low-fat diet and exercise do not change your cholesterol and triglyceride levels satisfactorily, you may need medication to do the job. The various cholesterol-lowering agents available decrease total and "bad" (LDL) cholesterol either by binding with cholesterol in the gastrointestinal tract (and eliminating it through the bowel) or by decreasing the amount of cholesterol produced by the liver.

Cholestyramine and *colestipol* bind in the gastrointestinal tract with the cholesterol-containing bile produced by the liver and eliminate it in the feces. While they are effective in lowering cholesterol levels, they frequently cause bloating, constipation, or nausea. These and other distressing side effects have limited their use to some degree.

Niacin is a vitamin which in high quantities decreases the manufacture of bad (LDL) cholesterol by the liver. It also raises good (HDL) cholesterol and lowers triglycerides. Unfortunately, niacin may cause frequent and uncomfortable flushing and stomach upset. It should not be taken in the presence of liver disease, diabetes, ulcers, or significant heart rhythm disturbances.

A second class of drugs is also available which lower cholesterol production by blocking a specific liver enzyme. In addition to helping lower bad (LDL) cholesterol, these drugs help increase good (HDL) cholesterol and decrease triglycerides. The two currently available agents, *lovastatin* and *pravastatin*, have a lower incidence of side effects than the other cholesterol-lowering drugs and are therefore widely used. However, they can occasionally cause liver abnormalities. This is easily detectable with blood tests and is reversible when the drug is stopped. Blood tests which measure liver injury need to be taken regularly in patients taking these agents.

Medications for Heart Failure

Heart failure is caused by a weakening of the ability of the heart to pump a sufficient output of blood to meet the body's needs. When this happens, a buildup of fluid in the lungs can occur, causing shortness of breath and frequently fluid buildup in the ankles and feet as well. Three types of drugs—diuretics, digitalis, and vasodilators—are currently available to treat this condition.

Diuretics. This group of drugs increase the amount of salt and water in the urine, thus decreasing the fluid in the lungs, ankles, and feet. This causes a significant decrease in shortness of breath and leg swelling. Because they are generally safe and effective, most physicians prescribe a diuretic as the first approach to treating heart failure. These agents are also effective in treating high blood pressure.

Diuretics have usually minor side effects. They do, however, wash potassium out of the body, and this loss can be dangerous if it is not corrected. Low body potassium can cause problems varying from mild leg cramps to serious heart rhythm disturbances. The best way to counteract the loss of potassium is to take potassium supplements, either food high in potassium, such as orange juice or bananas, or a potassium liquid or pill. A less common approach is to use a potassium-sparing diuretic, such as *spironolactone* or *triamterene*, weak as a diuretic but effective in preventing excess loss of potassium. Patients taking diuretics should have their blood potassium level measured on a regular basis. Other possible side effects of diuretics include stomach upset and skin rash.

Digitalis. Usually administered in conjunction with a diuretic drug, digitalis enhances heart muscle contraction and is effective also in controlling certain types of heart rhythm disturbances. While digitalis therapy can be helpful, the drug has potentially serious side effects (digitalis toxicity), among them dangerous heart rhythm disturbances. These occur most often in patients with advanced heart failure who are taking high doses of diuretics and have low potassium levels. Low potassium significantly increases the likelihood of digitalis toxicity. Therefore blood potassium levels and electrocardiograms of patients on this medication must be checked regularly.

Vasodilators. These agents, which dilate the blood vessels, have become important in the treatment of heart failure. The most effective among them are those which block an enzyme that converts a substance in the body called angiotensin. (The enzyme is called angiotensin-converting enzyme, and these drugs are known as ACE inhibitors.) They increase the efficiency of the weakened heart by decreasing the arteries' resistance to its pumping action. ACE inhibitors are most commonly used as a backup to diuretics and digitalis. However, they are increasingly being used early in heart failure management. They are also used to treat hypertension.

The major side effect is excessive lowering of the blood pressure. Careful monitoring of blood pressure levels is therefore crucial, particularly when the drug is first taken, so that a safe, correct dose can be determined. Vasodilators should not be taken by patients with kidney disease. Other, less frequent side effects include abnormal blood counts, allergic reactions, cough, and skin rash.

TAKING MEDICATION PROPERLY

• Understand the medications you are taking, and why. Ask your doctor:

What does the drug do? How does it work?

How is it going to help? Will it prolong life, prevent disease, decrease symptoms?

What are the possible risks or side effects? What warning signs are there?

Is there any risk of interaction with other substances?

• When you get a prescription filled, there is an enclosed package insert. This insert gives you more detail about the drug: its uses, dosages, *and* potential side effects. It is very important to *read this carefully*. Keep the package insert for future reference.

• Be sure you understand the correct way to take your medication—the precise dosage, number of pills, *and* the scheduled number of times each day. It helps to time your medication with other events; if you need to take a pill once daily, for instance, before bedtime or upon awakening works well. If the medication needs to be taken four times a day, once at each meal and at bedtime is a convenient schedule.

• If you forget to take your medication, do *not* take additional pills to make up for any you have missed. Simply go back on your original schedule.

• All drugs have potential side effects. If you think you may be experiencing any, do not stop taking the medicine. Call your doctor and discuss the problem.

• Do *not* stop taking your medicine because you are

feeling well. A medicine often is needed to control a problem that will recur if you stop treatment on your own. Certainly, you should feel free to discuss stopping any medicine with your doctor if it seems reasonable to you.

CHAPTER 12

Afterword: Where We Are, and Where We Are Going

The health concerns of women finally are being addressed nationally. Under the leadership of Dr. Bernadine Healy, the National Institutes of Health launched the Woman's Health Initiative to bridge serious gaps in knowledge about women's health. Members of Congress also have begun to encourage more studies on women's health.

However belatedly, doctors and researchers have recognized that cardiovascular disease is, to quote the American Heart Association, "an equal-opportunity killer." Critical questions urgently require answers: What is the role of estrogen replacement therapy in protecting women from heart disease? What is the relative importance of total cholesterol, good and bad cholesterol, and triglyceride levels in women? What constitutes a healthy diet for women? Are the risks and benefits of medications the same for women as for men? How can cardiac diagnostic tests be improved and risks involved in treatments such as bypass surgery be reduced?

Clinical trials are needed to provide answers to these and other questions about women and heart disease. One study, Postmenopausal Estrogen/Progestin Intervention (PEPI), the largest female-oriented clinical study in U.S. history, was launched recently by the NIH, and is evaluating 840 postmenopausal women aged forty-five to sixty-four, at seven medical centers across the country. Over the next several years, the effects of various estrogen-progestin combinations will be tested and their effects on cholesterol, blood sugar, blood clotting, and other factors that can influence a woman's risk of heart disease will be evaluated. Says Dr. Elizabeth Barrett-Connor, chair of the PEPI steering committee, "Heart disease is the single most common cause of death in both men and women. Until recently, the 'and women' was not appreciated."

The NIH has issued a directive to medical investigators seeking its financial support insisting that their research proposals specifically include female subjects. This will ensure that progress in fighting heart disease can apply to *all* Americans. I expect substantial progress in the next decade. New methods and a wide array of approaches will be found to halt and even reverse atherosclerosis—from healthy lifestyle changes and new medicines, to more sophisticated devices and techniques, such as lasers. Genetic engineering research will also result in important breakthroughs, as will research focused on how the power of the mind can be mobilized for health (this new field is called psychoneuro-immunology).

While medical research fills some gaps in knowledge, several aspects of heart health and the way to achieve it are quite clear today. The value of exercise for women is undeniable. Physical and mental reinvigoration, healthy weight maintenance, an increase in good cholesterol and decrease in stress are just a few of its benefits. Eating a low-fat diet (less than 30 percent of total calories from fat) and maintaining a healthy weight are also invaluable. There is a proven relationship among high-fat diet, obesity, and heart risk for women, and evidence is accumulating that the risk for cancer is likewise related. Learning to handle stress is essential for good health. Women feel stress today more than ever, and its effects on women's health are inarguable. And smoking is without doubt the number-one health hazard for women today. Despite repeated warnings about smoking, and despite findings that kicking the habit decreases the risks of heart disease and cancer dramatically, too many women continue to smoke.

Where does this leave you, the reader? How can you begin to decrease your risk of heart disease and improve the quality of your life at the same time? The single most important decision you can make in this regard is to take responsibility for your own health. This means first becoming knowledgeable about the vital matters discussed in this book and how they apply to you. The next step is to make a commitment to take good care of yourself and your body. Caring for others begins with caring for yourself and knowing you are worth it. Your commitment then can be translated into a specific plan of action which is flexible, realistic, and modifiable. Your goal is not perfection but consistency with your aim of good health by staying in alignment with that purpose. Without minimizing the challenges, I know you *can* do it and I support you fully. Remember that wonderful quote from Ecclesiastes, "There is a time for every purpose." Let your time be now.

Glossary

Adrenaline. A secretion of the adrenal glands (also called epinephrine) which constricts blood vessels and increases heart rate and blood pressure.

Aneurysm. A saclike bulging of the heart or a blood vessel due to weakening by disease, trauma, or birth defect.

Angiogram. An X-ray examination of the heart or blood vessels after a dye is injected into the bloodstream.

Angioplasty. A catheterization technique in which a balloon or other device (such as a laser) is used to dilate the obstructed artery.

Anti-anginal. A drug that relieves symptoms of angina pectoris.

Anti-arrhythmic. A drug that controls or prevents heart rhythm disturbances.

Anticoagulant. A drug that slows the clotting of blood, helps prevent new clots and enlargement of existing clots, and decreases the likelihood of embolism.

Antihypertensive. A drug that lowers blood pressure.

Aorta. The largest artery of the body, which originates from the heart and transports blood to its many arterial branches.

Arteriole. The smallest type of artery, which transports blood from the larger arteries to the capillaries.

Arteriosclerosis. Hardening of the arteries. A broad term applying to various conditions that cause the walls of arteries to thicken and lose their elasticity.

Atherosclerosis. A type of arteriosclerosis in which the artery wall is infiltrated by cholesterol and other materials. When these deposits enlarge, they project into the inner portion of the artery and obstruct the flow of blood.

Auscultation. The act of listening to the heart, lungs, and other parts of the body with a stethoscope.

Bacterial endocarditis. An inflammation of the inner layer of the heart, particularly its valves, caused by bacterial infection.

Capillary. A tiny vessel whose wall consists of a single layer of cells through which oxygen and nutrients move to the tissues of the body, and through which carbon dioxide and other waste products are transported from the tissues for elimination.

Cardiac. Pertaining to the heart. Also used to refer to someone with heart disease.

Cardiovascular. Pertaining to the heart and blood vessels.

Cardioversion. The restoration of a normal heart rhythm by means of an electrical shock applied across the chest.

Carotid arteries. The two vessels that provide blood to the right and left sides of the brain.

Catheter. A thin tube of plastic or other material. In cardiac catheterization, the tube is inserted into a vein or artery and advanced to the heart under X-ray guidance.

Cerebrovascular accident. A stroke: partial or total paralysis of a portion of the body due to brain malfunction brought on by vascular disease.

Claudication. Pain in the calf of one or both legs, usually while walking, due to obstructive disease of the arteries supplying the lower extremities.

Coagulation. The formation of a clot.

Collateral circulation. Blood vessels which originate as a result of a severely blocked artery and supply blood to a jeopardized area.

Coronary artery. A blood vessel on the surface of the heart which supplies it with oxygen and nutrients.

Coronary thrombosis. The formation of a clot on the inner surface of a damaged coronary artery, often results in a heart attack. The term sometimes is used to refer to a heart attack.

Dilatation. The enlargement or widening of the heart or blood vessels.

Diuretic. A drug that increases the amount of salt and water excreted by the urine.

Dyspnea. Difficult or labored breathing.

Edema. A swelling due to an accumulation of salt and water in the body.

Embolism. The obstruction of a blood vessel by a blood clot fragment (or other substance) which has broken off from the larger clot and traveled in the bloodstream to lodge elsewhere.

Epinephrine. A secretion of the adrenal glands which constricts blood vessels and increases heart rate and blood pressure.

Etiology. The cause of a disease.

Extrasystole. A premature heartbeat.

False negative test. A test yielding normal ("negative") results in a patient who actually has a disease.

False positive test. A test yielding abnormal ("positive") results in a patient who actually has no disease.

Fatty acid. A chemical unit of fat, which is saturated, unsaturated, or monounsaturated.

Femoral artery. The main artery supplying blood to the leg.

Fibrillation. A chaotic heart rhythm that causes the heart muscle to cease effective contraction. Atrial fibrillation, involving the atria, results in a decrease of 20 to 30 percent of heart output. Ventricular fibrillation, involving the ventricles, results in stopping all heart output.

Fibrinolytic. Having the ability to dissolve a blood clot.

Heart block. The partial or complete interruption of the heart's electrical impulse from the atria to the ventricles. People with this condition frequently require an artificial pacemaker.

Heart-lung machine. An apparatus that provides oxygen to blood diverted from the heart during open heart surgery.

Heparin. An anticoagulant which prevents blood from clotting and already existing clots from enlarging or breaking off.

Hypercholesterolemia. Excess cholesterol in the blood.

Hyperlipemia. Excess fat (lipid) in the blood.

Hypertension. High blood pressure.

Hypertrophy. An increase in amount of heart muscle mass.

Hypotension. Low blood pressure.

Hypoxia. Low oxygen level in the blood.

Interatrial septum. The wall of heart muscle between the right and left atria.

Interventricular septum. The wall of heart muscle between the right and left ventricles.

Ischemia. A temporary imbalance between the oxygen demand of a portion of the heart muscle and the oxygen supply provided by one or more obstructed coronary arteries.

Lipid. Fat.

Lipoprotein. A compound of fat and a protein that carries fats such as cholesterol through the bloodstream.

Lumen. The channel inside a blood vessel.

Monounsaturated fat. A type of fat that can absorb one hydrogen atom. Monounsaturates, among them olive oil, tend to be associated with lower cholesterol.

Murmur. A sound that can be heard with a stethoscope over the heart or an artery, attributable to turbulence of blood flow. Murmurs can be innocent (of no significance), or can indicate an abnormality, as of a cardiac valve.

Myocardial infarction. Damage of an area of heart muscle due to inadequate blood supply. A heart attack.

Myocarditis. An inflammation of the heart muscle, most commonly due to excess alcohol intake or a virus.

Myocardium. The heart muscle.

Open-heart surgery. An operation on the opened heart, during which blood is diverted through a heart-lung machine.

Pacemaker. 1. Referring to specialized cells of the heart that generate the electrical impulses which depolarize the heart muscle and cause it to contract. 2. An electrical device implanted in the heart to control its rate and rhythm when its natural pacemaker cells are defective.

Paroxysmal tachycardia. An episode of rapid heartbeat, which usually starts and stops suddenly.

Pathogenesis. The origin of a disease.

Percussion. A method of detecting disease by tapping the fingers over the lungs and other parts of the body.

Pericarditis. An inflammation of the pericardium, the sac surrounding the heart.

Phlebitis. An inflammation in a vein (often in the leg), which is accompanied by a blood clot.

Plaque. A buildup of cholesterol and other fatty deposits in an artery wall.

Plasma. The liquid portion of the blood with the blood elements removed in an uncoagulated state.

Prognosis. A prediction of the future outcome of a disease or condition.

Prophylaxis. Preventive treatment.

Psychosomatic. Referring to a disorder caused by the mind and emotions, and characterized by symptoms that mimic those of disease.

Pulmonary. Pertaining to the lungs.

Pulmonary edema. A severe form of heart failure in which substantial amounts of fluid collect in the lungs, causing severe shortness of breath.

Pulmonary embolism. The lodging of a blood clot (or fragment) in a pulmonary artery after breaking off from another clot, usually located in the legs.

Rheumatic heart disease. A condition due to damage to the heart valves from rheumatic fever, which develops as a reaction to streptococcal infection.

Saturated fat. A dietary fat that cannot absorb hydrogen. A diet high in saturated fat results in high blood cholesterol levels.

Sclerosis. A hardening.

Septum. A wall of heart muscle between chambers of the heart.

Serum. The fluid portion of the blood with the cell elements removed by coagulation.

Shock. A state caused by a failing circulation and characterized by low blood pressure, low urine output, and cold, clammy skin.

Shunt. An opening between two portions of the heart or two blood vessels, through which blood flow is diverted.

Spasm. A temporary constriction of an artery which narrows or occludes it.

Sphygmomanometer. An instrument that measures blood pressure.

Stasis. The stoppage or pooling of blood or other body fluid.

Stenosis. The narrowing of a heart valve or an artery.

Stethoscope. An instrument for listening to the heart, lungs, and other organs in the body.

Streptokinase. An agent that dissolves clots.

Stroke. A partial or total paralysis of a portion of the body due to the brain damage caused by vascular disease.

Syncope. A faint.

Syndrome. A set of symptoms due to a common cause.

Tachycardia. A rapid heart rate.

Thrombolytic. Able to dissolve clots; such an agent.

Thrombophlebitis. The inflammation and clotting of a vein (usually in the legs).

Thrombosis. The formation, development, or presence of a blood clot.

Tissue plasminogen activator (TPA). A clot-dissolving agent manufactured by genetic engineering.

Urokinase. An agent that dissolves clots.

Vascular. Pertaining to the blood vessels.

Ventricular premature beat. An early beat or contraction originating in the ventricles.

Very low-density lipoprotein (VLDL). Lipoprotein that carries cholesterol and triglycerides through the bloodstream.

Acknowledgments

Many people have been helpful in the shaping of this book. I thank in particular Linda Cohen, a very special friend, and Lucy Labson, a very special sister, for giving me a woman's perspective. I am grateful to Ralph Melarango for his insights and suggestions, and to Steve Hasenberg and Gerald Newmark for their valuable input. Gerald Jampolsky, M.D., offered me his unique perspectives and his encouragement, for which I am most appreciative. I am grateful also to Sue and Art Goldfarb, Jim Stein, Bud Lehman, Gary Gilson, Mark Fahanian, as well as Dr. Terry Binkovitz and Doreen Rivera. June Lockhart's comments and support were encouraging. A warm thank you to these cardiologists for sharing their professional opinions: Ronald Pennock, Lloyd Klein, David Williams, David Cannom, Richard Berger, and Robert Katz. In addition, I want to thank my children, Sharon and Steve, for giving me the vantage point of youth.

Last, I am in debt to Dan Green, my agent, and Jane Isay, my editor at Putnam, for their superb advice, enthusiastic ongoing encouragement, and warm friendship.

Index